SEXY *by* NATURE

The Whole Foods
Solution to
Radiant Health,
Lifelong Sex Appeal,
and Soaring Confidence

STEFANI RUPER

Victory Belt Publishing, Inc.
Las Vegas

For Dorothy

Table of Contents

Foreword

by J. J. Virgin

My client, looking exasperated, pointed to the endless containers of fat-free yogurt as we strolled through her local health-food store. "You mean to tell me I ate this nasty stuff that tastes like wallpaper paste for years and it's not even healthy?"

Within her reaction I heard equal parts frustration and joy: she realized that while manufacturers and so-called experts had misled her, she needn't ever again endure those awful-tasting health-food impostors.

If you're like most women I've worked with over my nearly three decades as a celebrity nutritionist and fitness expert, you've played by the rules, yet you struggle to get or stay lean and healthy. You've religiously followed the "healthy" nutrition guidelines: fat-free yogurt, low-fat cheese, artificial sweetener or agave in your "lite" latte, whole-grain "goodness," and soy everything.

That plan isn't working. It never worked. And it's not your fault.

It's not because you're genetically doomed or not working hard enough. You're a smart, focused woman who has simply followed the wrong set of guidelines.

Myth-buster is a role I frequently play in my job. Every time I start to think that we're headed in the right direction when it comes to understanding nutrition and optimal health, I read an article in a women's magazine by some so-called expert making some boneheaded, completely inaccurate assertion about what to eat or how to exercise.

Savvy manufacturers, eager to pimp their "healthy" foods, only add to the confusion as they profit financially even as your health takes a direct hit. It would be comical if the repercussions weren't so tragic. As our waistlines expand, so too do diabetes, heart disease, and other killers.

Being a myth-buster is a tiring, never-ending job. Thankfully, I'm not alone in this endeavor. In her new book, *Sexy by Nature,* Stefani Ruper tackles numerous nutrition fallacies that steal our sexy and sabotage our health. Among these are low-calorie diets, low-fat diets, vegetarian diets, soy-rich foods, and MyPlate (formerly known as the Food Pyramid). Any of those sound familiar? They don't work, they've never worked, and the only thing they've succeeded in doing is making us fat and sick.

So how *do* you eat? Well, Ruper shows you that, too, providing an easy-to-implement blueprint that incorporates a whole-foods, evolutionary approach that kept humans healthy, lean, and active for millennia. Your body will thrive on these same nutrient-rich, satisfying foods today and will stay lean and sexy for life.

Ruper combines science-based research with an informative, entertaining style that will help you put her strategies into action immediately. She takes all the guesswork out of becoming lean and healthy by telling you not only what to eat, but how, how much, and when. *Sexy by Nature* is like having a sassy, super-smart nutritionist take you gently but firmly by the hand and lead you to wiser decisions.

Any good health expert knows that optimal health goes beyond food. Hormonal imbalances, inflammation, stress, lack of sleep, and a wrecked metabolism all contribute to making you gain fat, making you feel lousy, and crashing your libido. Ruper tackles all these issues and provides a hands-on plan to help you look and feel more vibrant and sexy.

Ruper's underlying premise is that if you love your body, it will love you back. Sounds simple enough, yet why do so many women struggle with this idea? *Sexy by Nature* provides a no-nonsense, tough-love approach about how to love and nourish your body. No matter what your age or current condition, you have the tools to regain optimal health, vigor, and *joie de vivre.*

You needn't surrender to low libido, fatigue, crankiness, or that unflattering muffin top as you grow older. *Sexy by Nature* is a comprehensive, fun-to-read blueprint for optimal female health. Within these pages lies a powerful, effective set of rules to change your health and your life.

Introduction

What Is Sexy?

In 2012, *Maxim* magazine declared 39-year-old actress Sofia Vergara the sexiest woman alive. I remember the shock I felt when I read the article. I wasn't surprised that they found her physicality sexy—Vergara's hourglass shape puts the little timekeeper in my Pictionary box to shame—but I was caught off-guard by the rest of the magazine's reasons. *Maxim* emphasized Vergara's maturity, outrageous personality, sense of humor, and boldness as important reasons for finding her sexy. Society sometimes does things right, I thought. High-fives for everybody. I ended that day with a skip in my step and woke the next day refreshed from happy dreams.

This morning, I conducted a thorough Internet search to dig up that article. I wanted to start this book with a grand overture to the power of personality in Vergara's sex appeal. Even more importantly, I wanted to explore how her personality had won over even *Maxim's* male voters. That would be a lovely way to demonstrate the rich depth that underlies society's ideas about sex appeal, I thought. Why not give credit where credit is due? I sat down with Google at 7:45 a.m., and it is now 9:41. The closest thing I have found to what I remember reading is a quote Vergara gave to *Maxim* about never wanting to get a breast reduction. Not quite the inspirational pick-me-up I was looking for.

Obviously, there are a lot of things wrong with the way we do sexy these days. The idea of women as sex objects has been deeply ingrained in our consciousness for a very long time. This is not a good thing. It is, in fact, a Very. Bad. Thing. It dehumanizes us. It turns violence against us. It destroys our self-esteem and makes us compete with one another over the most trivial things. I hate the idea of women being sex objects with fiery passion—as much as, if not much more than, any other bra-burning feminist I know.

But I also know that our culture values more in the realm of sex appeal than it appears at first horrifying glance. It is the skin we live in, but not *just* the skin we live in. I *did* at some point read glorious reviews of Vergara's personality with regard to her sex appeal. I also know that Tina Fey was elected to the lists of the Top 99 Sexiest Women of 2012 by AskMen.com and the 50 Hottest Women on Television by Ugo.com. I know that millions of people defend Adele's sex appeal not just because of her heart-breaking melodies but also because of her fierce pride and empowered embodiment.

Think about the women and men in your life. Think about your own sexual desires. Think about when you feel sexy and when you do not. How much of it is about specific physical characteristics, and how much of it is about the way sexy people carry themselves, interact with others, and appear confident, comfortable, and alive in their own skin? How much of it is about talent, skill, smarts, or being a good person? How much of it is hard to articulate, but feels like a package deal in which the whole person is important?

Sexy isn't an hourglass figure. It isn't a swimsuit. It isn't a bra size or a hair color or the ability to fit into a tiny dress. It's none of these things, because none of these things puts fire in your eyes or fierce confidence in your stride. So what is sexy?

Sexy is an attitude. Sexy is empowerment. Sexy is excitement to be in the skin you're in.

This book shows you how to get there. I do so by walking you through a series of steps. Step 1 constitutes the strategy: it tears down the standard, outdated rules by which most people play the health and fitness game. These rules haven't done us any real service. In their stead, I lay out seven smart and efficient new rules by which I and millions of other happy, sexy women covertly live. These rules ask: what does the female body need to heal and become sexy all on its own?

Step 2 is about these needs as they apply to food. Which foods impede health and sexiness, and which are the natural power-houses the female body is designed to use for healing and weight loss? Step 3 details lifestyle factors, such as stress reduction and sun exposure, that also help provide female bodies with the stuff they need. Together, Steps 2 and 3 outline a powerful set of diet and lifestyle changes that will make you naturally more power-ful, healthy, energetic, and sexy every single day.

Step 4 is tailored to your own obstacles and desires. Have acne? Nature can make you radiant for good. Want a kick-ass li-bido? It'll naturally skyrocket. Struggle with PMS? Infertility? Weight loss? These problems are now a part of your past. No, the solutions to these problems are not immediate. There is no magic wand to wave. There is, however, real healing and real health on realistic timetables. And that's exactly what you need for perma-nent health. Step 4 explains how specific conditions can negatively affect female health and shows you how to naturally restore the health and vitality you were built for.

Step 5 ties everything together. While you will certainly feel and be sexier after completing Steps 2, 3, and 4, Step 5 gives you the emotional support, ideas, and practices to turn your inherent sexiness into a permanent and powerful feature of your life. You'll feel healthy and alluring. You'll develop a good relationship with your body. And you'll live out your life with the fiery passion and delight of a healthy, embodied, and radiantly alive woman.

Is my way the only way to do it? Of course not. Is it the best way? Absolutely it is.

I have developed these methods after years of seeking, think-ing, and living. They come from years of research, blogging, and networking. They come from working with thousands of women across the globe. They come from my childhood home in Detroit and from my adult life on the East Coast and in China, Italy,

France, Taiwan, and Indonesia, where I have been a student, a writer, a philosopher, a go-go dancer, and a woman who walks down the street every day and looks strangers in the eye with a smile.

What makes me feel my best? What makes the whole community of women feel our best? What best provides the basis for a long life of good health in which you feel great about yourself? Nature does. Harmony with your body does. Positivity, pride, and love do. The methods I deliver in this book will help you reach all these goals with radical efficiency and long-lasting effects.

My story
and
Why You Need This Book

In the fall of 2009, my jean size dropped from ten to double zero over the course of just three months. I was not the only one who noticed. Approximately once a week, one of my friends drew the short straw and had me over for dinner. She'd lean across the dinner table, hold my hand, let her eyes well up, and tell me (again) that she was concerned I had a *problem*.

"Screw this!" I scoffed. I laughed, and often. I had never felt better about myself. I had been trying to ditch my love handles for ten years, and finally I had shed them. Hallelujah! Men looked at me differently. Eyes wandered up and down my body, and smiles followed. An old love interest who had spurned me began pursuing me relentlessly. I tried on fancy dresses at the mall and compared myself to supermodels. Life could not have been any better.

I did not understand why my friends thought I had a problem. I did everything the way I was told. My professors made it quite clear that the healthiest thing to be was a vegetarian, so I stopped eating animals. Talk show hosts proclaimed loudly that fat was unhealthy, so I didn't eat it. Celebrity magazines made it obvious that I had to be thin to be sexy, so I measured my waistline every night. My doctor's office had a chart with the body mass index on it and smiley faces toward the lower end, so I drove my BMI downward. Medical professionals equated low-calorie diets with better health, so I went to sleep hungry every night. Much as my friends thought I had a problem, I was playing the game the way it was supposed to be played. I followed all the rules. It just so happened that I was doing it well enough to *win*.

I might have felt differently about winning the game if I had listened at all to my own body. I stopped menstruating. I became infertile. I was diagnosed with polycystic ovarian syndrome, hypothyroidism, and hypothalamic amenorrhea. I lost all vestiges of a sex drive. I obsessed over food and constantly felt deprived. I did not eat enough to give my body the nutrients it needed. I developed a nasty case of acne, and I worked out hard for at least 90 minutes every day, usually twice a day. That was how I *lived*. I thought that was what I had to do to in order to win.

Several months later, I packed up and wandered across the globe. I lived in Venice. There, I flirted my way onto Mediterranean yachts. I backpacked around Europe and winked my way into sold-out concerts. I went to school in Taichung, Taiwan. When a bar owner noticed how much more fun his customers had when I danced on top of his bar rather than his usual go-go dancers, he hired me to do it instead. I was brashly confident, daringly open, and thrilled to be so free and alive.

"Winning" was working.

I couldn't go all the way around the world without coming home with a couple of lessons, however. Most importantly, I learned that how sexy I both *felt* and was *perceived to be* had everything to do with my confidence and very little to do with the shape my tiny body. Sure, my figure mattered in the eyes of other people. I looked more stereotypically fit than I used to. But I am willing to bet my life that had I acted the same self-assured, flirtatious way while having fat on my thighs, hips, and anywhere else, I would have received the same awe, had the same fun, and laughed just as joyously with the men and women I met in every location I wandered. Sexy was largely about *confidence,* and I could no longer ignore the fact that I sacrificed a lot in order to win for reasons that were becoming less and less clear.

This was somewhat bad news, because the hidden truth was that I had a confidence problem. Instead of being founded on love and loyalty to my body, my flirty confidence was completely dependent on how I looked. My happiness was, too. When I walked down the street, I met people's eyes and smiled on the days I felt thin and fit, and I looked down and off to the side on "fat" days. I had no real love, no real confidence, and no real allegiance to my body. I was tethered to how it looked to other people. Compared to image, I cared very little about my body's health, its inherent worth, or its glorious powers to move, dance, eat, sing, and live. When it came to having a strong and happy relationship with my body, I was Failing with a capital F.

What's more, my poor body was starving.

When I am interviewed on podcasts these days, people often ask me when I got started on the diet that I prescribe in this book. Even though I changed the basis of my diet to *Sexy by Nature* foods back in 2009, I now know and inform my listeners that it was not until years afterward that I actually developed the *Sexy by Nature* approach to wellness. This is because this "diet" is not only about the food you eat, but also, and perhaps more importantly, about the loving and nourishing way you do it.

The birth of a paradigm

It was a long road of research and experience before I figured out exactly what I needed other than whole foods in order to be healthy, happy, and free. First, I had to learn my way inside and out of the female reproductive and endocrine systems. Hypothalamic amenorrhea, anterior pituitary gland, Hashimoto's thyroiditis, and interleukin-6 became some of several hundred new words in my vocabulary. I studied vitamins, minerals, and foods as they might affect these systems. I did so in an effort to cure myself of my low libido, acne, and infertility, but I did not find the trick that would enable me to remedy these indicators of poor health while maintaining my low weight and restrictive lifestyle. I began to suspect that relaxing my grip on my image and developing a more natural, intuitive way of eating might be crucial to resolving my PCOS and other hormone problems. But I didn't want to do that. My last, desperate lunge at having my cake and eating it, too, was to experiment with pharmaceutical methods. The drugs I took set in motion eighteen months of panic attacks. That was the straw that broke the camel's back. I might have been willing to suffer a low libido in order to be thin, but I would not let myself destroy my mental health. No longer could I continue to do what I had been doing to myself for years. In one liberating yet terrifying week, I threw my rabid body perfectionism out the window and never looked back. I was finally on my body's side, and for good.

Around the same time I was learning all these things about my body's need for nourishment, I started to think about my destructive behaviors on a broader scale. What about all the other women in the world who suffered under the same norms and pressures? What about the preteen who starves herself to death, the new mother who is terrified of her post-birth body, or the near 80 percent of young women who have negative body image issues? What about all the beautiful young girls being born into this twisted, restrictive, objectifying culture? Of all the things I did in this period, the most important is what I did next.

I got *angry*.

And thus my website and community were born.

And thus this life-changing manifesto was born. *Sexy by Nature* contains lessons I learned while studying the female body and wandering the globe—lessons that thousands of women have since come to love and internalize and live by. Sexy is not restriction. Sexy is not discipline. Sexy is not thin. Sexy is not meeting someone else's expectations. Sexy is about fitness and having a strong, shapely, feminine figure particular to your own genes and your own nature. Sexy is being excited to be at home in your own body. Sexy is having such a good relationship with your body that no amount of magazine ads taunting you will ever put you at war with yourself again. I am firmly on the side of my body now. I know that being healthy is what makes me sexy. My body is a natural body that needs me to listen to it and love it and nourish it. The more I give it these things, the sexier I am and the better my life gets. The more I give my body love, the more my body loves me back. Clear skin. Better sleep. A ravenous libido. A naturally maintained sexy waistline. Positive mental energy. Energy to set the world on fire.

This is where the *Sexy by Nature* Golden Rule comes into play.

The *Sexy by Nature* Golden Rule

Your body is a natural body with natural needs that, when loved properly, loves you right back.

This book is for you because your body has the same natural ability that mine has to be sexy and healthy all on its own. It naturally slims itself, naturally heals itself, and naturally generates feelings of peace and happiness. All your body needs is for you to work *with* it rather than against it. All it needs is the natural nourishment it has been craving all along.

If you play by the *Sexy by Nature* Golden Rule and love and nourish your natural body, then you will join me on the road to radical, easy, and healthy sex appeal.

The Nature Rules that I outline in Step 1 are about standing up for yourself and your body in the face of everything in the world that tells you otherwise. It can be a challenge for sure. Saying no to processed foods and putting away diet magazines... these are big steps for a lot of us. Revolutions, even. But worth it? Unquestionably. I am with you every step of the way. And in the end, loyalty to living this way is the easiest thing in the world. When you give your body what it needs to be sexy all under its own power—without drugs or doctor's visits or side effects or degenerative disease—health is not a struggle. Being sexy is not a struggle. Being at home in your own skin is not a struggle. It's a journey in life and in love, and an electrifyingly sexy one at that.

1: Trailblaze

> *"Don't play the game,*
> *beat the game."*
>
> —TIM FERRISS

If there is anything universally true about health today, it's that we have forgotten how to do it. As of 2012, nearly 240 million Americans are overweight. Approximately 120 million are obese, and 26 million have diabetes.[1] At any given time, 20 percent of Americans say that they are on a diet.[2] That's almost 50 million people, and millions more are not following a specific diet but are embroiled in a lifelong struggle for health and weight loss. We are sick, and we are fat, and it doesn't look like we will be getting better anytime soon.

It's not our fault that we have failed. In this culture, we are entrenched in a game that was rigged against us from the start. Food has been designed to make us addicted to it. The pharmaceutical industry has a vested interest in keeping us sick—it pays the bills. Science is conducted with the biases of old habits and monetary interests in mind. Nutrition standards are in the hands of lobbyists. Popular media has exploited women as objects and deployed an aggressive offense against self-esteem and self-love. Worse, perhaps, we as a people have developed a set of rules about how to navigate these institutions that are restrictive, punitive, encouraging of self-loathing, and antagonistic to physical health. How can we achieve real and lifelong health and weight loss? Not by following these rules.

"Don't play the game, beat the game," says entrepreneur Tim Ferriss. We have the option to play. We could listen to the food industry. We could take drugs. We could starve ourselves to lose weight. We could become low-fat vegetarians. Are these good ideas? Not by my estimation. My own experience with the Standard American Diet (SAD) and what I call the Standard

American Game (because it is in reality about so much more than just diet) led me to experience psychological and physical health horrors that I wouldn't wish on my worst enemies. The game as it's usually played involves more struggle, frustration, confusion, alienation, self-doubt, low self-esteem, and poor health than can ever be rightfully expressed.

Tim says one more thing I like: "Make the rules that change the rules." Life is too short to be a follower. So why not say no to struggle and failure and do things the smart way?

Try as I did to articulate a manifesto that stands on its own, I failed. In the end, I could not for the life of me write a book glorifying natural sexiness without devoting a significant chunk of it to tearing down the wretched old rules. For this reason, this chapter is divided into comparisons between the Old and the New. The Bad and the Good. The Ugly and the Lovely. What rules have led us so devastatingly far off-track? What's wrong with the Standard American Game, and how can we step outside these rules to beat this game? What can we learn from nature that aligns us with our bodies and provides us with real, enduring health?

Old rules and new rules in 60 seconds or less

The old rules are shrouded in ignorance, complacency, and pain. They entail harsh asceticism and self-deprivation and force you to work *harder* to achieve your health goals. The better alternative is to work *smarter*. The old rules lead to dependence on pharmaceutical companies; the smart alternative is to empower yourself to heal underlying problems. The old rules take the immense power of the female body for granted; the smart thing is to embrace your femaleness and use it to your advantage. In all these cases and more, I have taken what's unnatural and hurtful about the current norms and transformed them into smart, effective principles of nature, replacing negativity, hate, ignorance, and fear with knowledge, empowerment, peace, and love.

Old Rule #1:
Beauty conformity

As a woman living in modern Western culture, you have surely experienced pressure to conform to body image norms at some point. You saw a magazine. You went to a mall. You hung out with your girlfriends. How does it feel to think that your body needs to look a certain way in order to be beautiful? Downright awful, at least in my experience.

Allowing body image norms to permeate your conscious is the first Old Rule that needs to be done away with. It can make you resent your body, make you feel uncomfortable in your own skin, and put you at war with your very self.

When we try to fit into shapes, sizes, and looks that are unnatural for us, we usually end up trying to rigidly control our bodies. We become easily frustrated. We might hate our bodies. On far too regular a basis, women confess to me that they fantasize about slicing fat off of their hips with a knife. Or that they envy starving children across the globe because being overweight isn't an issue for them.

Even if your body size and body mass index are healthy, the pressure is tremendous. Almost every woman in the Western world labors day in and day out (sometimes unknowingly) to protect her self-esteem against external pressure. You are told to look a certain way, to fit a certain mold, to be perfect, and are deliberately made to feel so bad about yourself that purchasing clothing and cosmetics is the only solution to being beautiful. You are forced to idealize a body type that is not your natural body type. This wins a lot of people a lot of money.

Idealizing an unrealistic and unnatural body type is not just mentally unhealthy but also physically unhealthy. Women often undertake unhealthy diets and restrictive practices in wild attempts to achieve the unachievable. One example is the grapefruit diet, which is exactly what it sounds like: you are permitted to eat grapefruit and almost nothing else. A seemingly more innocent version is the one that I undertook back in 2009: vegetarian, low-fat, and low-calorie. Is such a diet good for the female body? No, it's not. The female body is uniquely sensitive to starvation signals and can turn to panic mode if those signals are detected. Starving yourself is not going to give you long-term health or sex appeal.

Perhaps worst of all is the fact that beauty norms pit women against each other. If I don't believe in the beautiful diversity of female bodies, I am constantly comparing myself to others. I measure myself, weigh myself, and judge myself. I always worry that I won't measure up. In turn, I measure others, weigh others, and judge others. I look at other women with narrowed, calculating eyes. I pit myself against them. I envy them. Is that woman sexier than I am? How do I get what she's got? Looks have become a competition. But if we reject the idea of a common, ideal body type and instead take pride in our own unique shapes, then we don't have to vie against each other in the race for beauty and love. We can, instead, celebrate our differences.

Nature Rule #1:
Celebratory uniqueness

Contrary to the airbrushed bodies plastered all over billboards and magazines, nature has made each of us a unique woman. This almost goes without saying, I know. But it's so important that I could write it a million times over. Society's addiction to conformity is nonsensical. This is especially the case once we acknowledge a basic truth of nature: you have a unique string of DNA, a unique body, a unique personality, and a unique story and life.

You have the option of chasing society's notion of an ideal body, but what good will that do you in the end? The science is crystal clear on this point: the more you try to fit your body into an unnatural shape, the less healthy you will be. The more you adhere to external notions of beauty, the fewer resources you have available to you to help you love yourself as you are.

Celebrating the unique beauty with which you were born does not mean that you cannot set goals. It does not mean that you give up on weight loss, fitness, clear skin, or any of the other external markers of health and sex appeal. Those are important, and this book is explicit about helping you work through them. It means only that you embrace your body as it has been designed. Nature Rule #1 says to throw totalizing rules out the window and stand allied with all women against them.

Nature Rule #1 makes you sexy because

it is sexy to own your natural self. It is sexy to be at peace with who you are. It is sexy to love yourself, and it is sexy to proudly have your own standards. It is sexy to walk with your chin up. The sexiest thing of all is to unashamedly be *you*.

This rule also makes you sexy because it empowers you to love and to be unafraid of other women. Without this fear, you can become confident, loving, and unwary of judgment from other women and men. When you do not fear other women, you can more easily love them (and they you!) and be friendly, open, smiling, flirtatious, and fun.

On nature, being you, and makeup

One of the most important tenets of this book is that the sexiest thing you can possibly be is yourself. In a book about appreciating natural womanhood, it might be easy to confuse my message with one that demands you eschew modern-day luxuries, fashion, and makeup. But this could not be further from the truth.

Do makeup and beauty products pose health risks? Not significant ones, and especially not if you opt for the natural, organic kinds that are free of laboratory chemicals.

None of the ideas in this book preclude you from wearing makeup, putting on fancy clothes, or owning 600 pairs of shoes. Go wild, I say! Do what makes you feel alive in your own skin. The only opinion I firmly hold on this score is that you do not *need* makeup to be beautiful. You do not *need* to be fashionable. You do not *need* facelifts or expensive jewelry or whatever *Vogue* tells you will make you beautiful this season. All you need is to embrace who you are and to live into that personality as fully and vibrantly as possible, inclusive of any makeup, clothing, and behaviors you choose to embrace.

Old Rule #2:
Restriction

Long before you or I arrived on this planet, America was a place where restriction ruled. Hedonism and gluttony certainly have their place in American culture, don't get me wrong; we need look no further than the orgy of chocolate bars at every checkout line. But the most *moral,* and therefore the most *good,* individuals have historically been the ones who abstained from bodily pleasures. The best Americans have always oriented their lives around piety, hard work, and discipline.

I am thinking specifically of the Puritans. Bear with me for a second—this is relevant. The Puritans came to America seeking religious freedom. Most of us know this part of the story well. What isn't normally taught in fourth-grade classrooms, however, is that the Puritans were so desperate to come here because they desired a lifestyle that denied all pleasure. They landed in the New World and immediately got to work painting the world in drab colors and living out self-flagellating, restrictive lives.

This legacy of self-denial comes to us from people other than the Puritans, too. For one thing, it lives in the Western religious tradition at large. Monks, nuns, and saints are idolized in Western culture in large part because they sacrifice physical pleasure.

This isn't to cast any sort of judgment on these types of religious lives. To the contrary. Asceticism can be a great and honorable value to embrace. I bring this up only to demonstrate how deeply rooted restriction is in the American psyche. American culture respects, honors, and reveres those who are able to give things up. Good things often go hand in hand with sacrifice.

Asceticism and women

Asceticism in the Western world is especially potent for women. Forgoing another history lecture, it goes almost without saying that women have long been forced into restrictive rituals and roles. One quick example is the role fasting has played in women's lives. Ever since the Middle Ages, women have fasted at rates far greater than men and to much more extreme degrees. Back then, fasting was thought to purify a woman, make her morally worthy, and enable her to develop a strong relationship with Jesus by mimicking his sacrifices. In medieval Europe, fasting was one of the only means by which women could achieve any level of goodness or experience the divine.

To get a feeling for how this practice has persisted into modern times, consider what you know of the means by which women typically pursue health in America today, and which of those health efforts earn applause from friends. For example, how many women do you know who go to the gym? And if they go often, do they get reverent oohs and aahs from their friends? Especially if they spend a lot of time there? "You must be in such great shape going to the gym twice a day! I could never do that. Wow!"

Another important question: how many of the vegetarians you know are women? According to a survey conducted by *Vegetarian Times* in 2008, about 3 percent of American adults are vegetarian, and 59 percent of them are women.[3] That's 150 percent the number of men. How often do vegetarians get those special oohs and aahs? I can't tell you how frequently people made me feel ecstatic by expressing awe for my vegetarianism back when I was playing the Standard Game. I couldn't get enough of their praise.

Ascetic:

1) Practicing strict self-denial as a measure of personal and especially spiritual discipline.

2) Austere in appearance, manner, or attitude.

The modern world's obsession with restriction has led to a wide variety of practices that are detrimental to health. These practices may masquerade as healthy, but they are not. Excess exercise is one of them. Fasting is another. Examples that might be harder to believe but are equally harmful include low-calorie diets, low-fat diets, and vegetarianism. This fact is made all the more unfortunate because these practices are especially harmful for women.

The farce of low-calorie dieting

One of the biggest problems facing us today is how obsessed we are with calories. This point is easy to demonstrate: as I write this, President Obama is signing into law a mandate that all restaurant chains publicize the calorie content of foods on their menus. It is possible, though not proven, that this practice will reduce calorie intake for some individuals. But will it actually make people healthier? What does the number of calories in a food say about the kind of nutrition it provides? Nothing. Calories convey *not a lick* about how healthy a food is.

Limiting calories for health and weight loss usually does more harm than good. Calories *do* matter, but they can't be the top priority. There are three main reasons why:

1. The nutrient status of a food has nothing to do with how many calories are in it. This idea contradicts standard nutritional advice in the Western world, which consistently conflates low-calorie foods with health, but it is nonetheless true. You can just as easily be nourished by high-calorie foods as you can by low-calorie foods. Coconut products are good examples of healthy high-calorie foods—and they might be one of the best defenses against Alzheimer's disease. Macadamia nuts, butter, and avocados are some others. On the other hand, the body can be significantly damaged by low-calorie foods. One great example is diet soda. In this case, "zero-calorie" is just a euphemism

for "nothing but chemicals." Even natural examples of low-calorie foods demonstrate how little power calories have. Celery is a natural low-calorie food that offers very little in the way of nutrition, especially when compared to higher-calorie and extremely nutrient-dense foods such as eggs. Calories convey energy content, not nutrient content. If you want to lose weight, calories can be a part of the equation, but fixing a broken metabolism by eating healthy foods should be your primary concern.

2. The body creates fat cells when it detects a calorie input that is too low. Once created, these fat cells *never go away.*

3. Low-calorie dieting leads to feelings of restriction and deprivation. Increased fat cell count may make it harder for dieters to stay lean, but a far more insidious effect of food restriction is the behavior that results from being deprived. Deprivation leads to extreme cravings, which lead to overeating. This, in turn, causes self-doubt and self-loathing. Self-doubt and self-loathing lead to even more restriction, which again causes extreme cravings and overeating. This cycle goes on and on, sometimes for decades. As such, restriction makes it nearly impossible to eat intuitively, to lose weight, or to be naturally healthy and slim. I cannot emphasize how harmful low-calorie thinking and eating is. It's just one of many aspects of the bad food rules, but it is woven into the fabric of just about every discussion on health in America.

The farce of low-fat dieting

America's love of asceticism has created distrust in a lot of things. Hearty meals have been some of the hardest hit, especially for women. Think about what a "healthy" woman might order at a restaurant versus what a healthy man would order: the man might order a steak, but the woman would likely have a salad with grilled chicken breast, and with the dressing on the side. Our obsession with restriction has given us a primal fear of all things hearty, fatty, and rich.

When American health began its precipitous decline in the latter half of the twentieth century, few authorities blamed the real culprits, such as sugar and processed foods. Instead, policymakers relied on ascetic intuitions about hearty meals and blamed higher-calorie, richer foods. This is an interesting phenomenon because hearty meals had been around for ages and people never got sick or fat. Processed foods, snack foods, and the incessant barrage of unnatural foods, however, were brand-new. Why didn't anyone point fingers at those products?

Fat in and of itself doesn't cause disease and weight gain. There are some unhealthy varieties of fat that do, but so do certain unhealthy carbohydrates. Trans fats are bad (as fats), and high-fructose corn syrup is bad (as a carbohydrate). It's not *fat* that's to blame for the health crisis; it is the *quality* of the fat and the *quality* of the carbohydrate that are to blame.

Extremely low-fat diets can be quite harmful. Why? First, because they cause an overreliance on unhealthy carbohydrates, which can cause weight gain and diabetes, among many other diseases of inflammation and poor metabolic health; and second, because fat is necessary for health and wellness. Fat comprises a significant portion of the contents of our cells, particularly the cell walls, as well as many of the important tissues in the body, such as brain and skin tissue. Without adequate fat intake, mental health weakens. Skin becomes dry and brittle. Cellular walls lose their integrity. Perhaps worst of all for women, hormone production is significantly impaired. Without fat, you can lose aspects of your fertility, your clear skin, your libido, and your femininity. Extremely low-fat diets do women a serious injustice, and for no reasonable justification that I can discern.

The farce of vegetarianism

Of all the old rules in this book, vegetarianism is the one that truly drives me up the wall. It doesn't make scientific sense, for one. Studies such as the China Study that in earlier decades "proved" vegetarianism to be the healthiest diet have since been shown to lack statistical significance.[4] Why do we continue to latch onto vegetarianism, then? There are a variety of reasons, some more valid than others. I wholeheartedly respect those who choose to forgo animal consumption for the sake of animal rights, sustainability, or religion. With respect to health, however, Western culture could not be more misguided. What usually happens is that a study is conducted and then the authors, journalists, or bloggers interpret the data to mean more than it should. For example, I once read a study that decried meat consumption because it showed that meat consumption was associated with poor blood cholesterol levels, but the "meat" that people in this study ate was pizza with meat on it. Not *natural meat,* but *pizza with meat on it.* This introduces several new variables, such as refined flour, processed cheese, processed meat, and what happens to the body when these things are eaten in combination. For this reason, these data cannot in any meaningful way influence our opinions on the health status of natural meat products. The only thing they can say is that eating pizza with meat on it is correlated with higher cholesterol levels.

Animal products are *crucial* for health. They are the only foods that contain vitamin B_{12}, a nutrient that people would die without. In fact, vegan parents in Alabama were recently convicted of murder after their infant died from B_{12} deficiency. Because of this risk, vegans need to supplement with B_{12}, or they'll die. Vegetarians must be careful and eat a lot of eggs or dairy products so that they get the B_{12} required for survival. If nothing proves that humans need to eat meat as a part of our very nature, this fact does. Other crucial vitamins that are abundant in animal products but not in plants include vitamin A (not beta-carotene, the plant-based precursor to vitamin A), choline, heme iron, and the omega-3 fatty acid DHA.

Yet as a culture we continue to conflate vegetarianism with greater health. Some people even go so far as to assert that vegetarianism is the most natural human diet. How can that be the case when it eschews vitamins that are crucial for health and wellness? When without animal products, infants die? It cannot. Our need for iron, zinc, copper, vitamin E, the rest of the B vitamins, and complete protein are other excellent reasons to eat meat.

For four years I ate a vegetarian diet. I became a vegetarian partly for the environment, and also for animal rights reasons. I now know, however, that there is at least one perfectly moral way to consume meat: with local, organic agriculture, which provides animal products that have been naturally and happily raised in fields of grass. Obtaining my meat from these sources enables me to meet my natural dietary needs while remaining in sync with my commitment to sustainability and environmental responsibility.

Health is too hard

Equally deleterious to American health as undertaking these scary ascetic practices is throwing one's hands up and saying, "No way, health looks like torture!" For every overweight person who restricts, diets, and continues to fail, there's another one who doesn't even try because health looks to them like such a sacrificial buzzkill.

People give up on the quest for good health for a wide variety of reasons. I have never seen one as powerful, however, as sacrifice. If you have to give up meat, give up fat, give up meals, and give up being satisfied by food in order to be healthy, it's going to be a hell of a lot harder to marry yourself to your quest. If you have to fast, or exercise all day every day, or become a *runner,* for goodness' sake, how is that going to make you feel about health?

The great news, however, is that you do not have to do any of those things.

The *Sexy by Nature* diet has nothing to do with restriction and everything to do with hearty meals and filling yourself up and being *satisfied*. In my experience, this principle of nourishment is not just *okay* but *necessary*. You *need* to eat to hearty satisfaction in order to get your body the nutrients it needs. *Sexy by Nature* says yes to all foods that are natural and nourishing. No number of calories, no amount of fat, and no amount of animal products is out of bounds.

Nature Rule #2:
Nourishment

The cornerstone of my approach to health lies in one simple commandment:

**Above and against all rules, nourish yourself.
When in doubt, choose nourishment.**

American culture is obsessed with restriction. I pointed out with respect to Old Rule #2 that this is largely because of how much we love asceticism. Yet it is probably caused by another factor as well: the modern world veritably *swims* in excess. We eat so gluttonously that it seems obvious that the answer is to do the opposite. That's not horrible reasoning. Instead of eating more, as we so often do, and so often become sick from doing, we should probably eat less, right?

The flaw in this logic comes from thinking that the *quantity* of food we eat is the problem. It's not. The real problem is the *quality* of food we eat. Most of the Standard American Diet has very little nutrition in it. The processed foods that comprise the SAD are devoid of the stuff that promotes healing and metabolic fitness and full of the stuff that blocks healing and decimates metabolic fitness. For this reason, the SAD makes us sick. The fact that we eat so much only exacerbates the underlying quality problem.

Bodies are designed to eat better foods than those found in the Standard American Diet. This is a pretty intuitive idea. It also happens to be backed up by solid science across a wide variety of fields. When the body's needs for nourishment aren't met, things go wrong. When they are met, things go right. It really is that simple. There's no

> Bodies are designed to eat better foods than those found in the Standard American Diet.

natural reason to deprive yourself of what your body needs. It *needs* nourishment. It needs vitamins and minerals and protein and fat and animal products. It needs calories. It does not need poor-quality foods. It does not need to be starved. It does not need to live off of celery sticks and zero-calorie dressing.

When you focus on nourishment, you satisfy your body. You feel sated and at peace, unlike so many of our low-calorie and vegetarian friends. Much of hunger, in fact, comes from nutrient deficiencies. When you don't feed your body the stuff that it was designed to eat, it remains hungry. The same goes for your psychological self. Instead of constantly depriving yourself of food and feeling so restricted and hungry, focus on nourishing your body and giving it healthy natural food, and you will leave food-related emotional distress in the dust.

Nourishment demands that you eat heartily. It gives you free rein to eat large meals. You can eat fat. You can eat animal products. You can eat carbohydrates. You can eat virtually any kind of food you want as long as it does not contain toxins. Focusing on nourishment is simultaneously the most fun and the healthiest thing you can do for your body. The more you focus on nourishing your body, the more free you are, and the more you heal.

Nourishment also facilitates listening. Whereas restrictive mentalities may compel you to ignore your body's natural signals, focusing on nourishment provides a platform for you to listen to your body and give it what it is asking for. It takes some time to learn the shapes of these different desires and to distinguish the unhealthy cravings from the healthy, nourishing ones, but these skills do come in time, facilitating an organic, happy relationship between you and your body.

Nature Rule #2 makes you sexy because

it makes you healthy inside and out. Nourishment gives you the physical goods you need to heal. It also gives you the psychological goods you need to develop a healthier, non-obsessive relationship with food and a more harmonious, respectful, and loving relationship with your body.

Old Rule #3:
Punishment

Old Rule #3 is the nasty partner in crime to Old Rule #2. As we value restrictive practices, so we also value discipline. And so we are hard on ourselves. And punish ourselves. "Harder, faster, stronger, leaner, better," we chant. "I should have been more," I used to tell myself approximately every eight seconds. "I could have been more. I could have *done* more. I didn't do enough. I need to do more. I've gotta get it right this time. I *need* to get it right this time."

Sound familiar?

Discipline is all well and good. I like it. I use it a lot. Finishing this book, for example, required more discipline than I ever knew I had. Discipline is a requirement for an enormous set of good practices. Hell, discipline is necessary in order to follow even *Sexy by Nature*'s easy guidelines. But when you couple discipline with asceticism or with punishment, then you have dumped yourself into a pile of physical and psychological trouble.

* * *

A lot of women are perfectionists. Even if we are not explicitly perfectionist, I'd argue that the majority of us come close to it. This is true at least insofar as we women are so tough on ourselves, especially with respect to our bodies, the way we look, and the diet and lifestyle practices we follow with respect to those things. Self-disciplined and self-punishing women comprise somewhere in the neighborhood of several dozen million women in the Western world, in my estimation. This is not a number to sneeze at.

The vast majority of the work I did consulting women, networking, and blogging over the last several years always came back to this issue. Almost none of the women I worked with knew how to forgive themselves. Few knew how to accept themselves. Few knew how to love themselves. Even fewer gave themselves the same kind of unconditional love and forgiveness that they gave their sisters, daughters, mothers, and friends. Almost none of us know how to escape the trap of self-punishment. It has sinisterly woven itself into the fibers of American femininity.

Today's world is a world of doubt. I grew up doubting myself. I compared myself to others. I was my own worst critic, bar none. This resulted in torturous self-punishing behaviors, such as spending hours at the gym every day or forbidding myself from eating for certain periods of time—none of which panned out in the long run. Even though disciplined behavior was supposed to get me back on track, it only made me feel worse about myself and more deprived. I felt alien in my body. I felt less like a natural, harmonious woman and more like a warrior in a never-ending battle against myself. I find it quite likely that this is case for millions of other women, too. Nearly every woman I have spoken with has experienced some degree of pressure to be hard on herself.

Nature Rule #3:
Love

What justification do we have for being hard on ourselves? None.

As far as I can tell, I punished myself out of fear. I was afraid of failing. I was afraid of gaining weight. I was afraid of not being sexy, of not being attractive, and of not being loved. I feared these things so desperately that I did everything I could conceive of to prevent them from happening. Setting high standards for performance was one of those things. If I was hard enough on myself, then there was no way I could fail. If I was disciplined enough, strong enough, or good enough, then I *had* to succeed.

The problem with this reasoning is twofold. First, punishment is not the best way to motivate yourself to do things. Psychologists know this well: punishment almost inevitably leads to negative behavior in the long run. A much better way to promote consistently good behavior is to use positive reinforcement. This is a fact of human nature, and a lesson we should take from the natural world.

I have rigorously applied this principle to my life and to the *Sexy by Nature* paradigm. It sits at the core of what this book is about. The less I punish myself, the easier it is to eat healthfully. Achieving good health, energy, weight loss, and clear skin is also easier. The less I punish myself, the less stressed I feel, and the healthier I am. It really is that simple.

My good behavior gives me positive rewards in the form of health benefits. This works so well that these days, punishment seems like the most ludicrous and harmful thing I could do for the sake of my health. Why get upset about the past? I have to forgive myself and move on. I have no other choice: positivity is the only way to improve my health and my happiness. If I punished myself, I'd increase my likelihood of failing and of engaging in negative, unhealthy behavior. Harsh discipline and punishment are counterproductive when it comes to making positive changes.

Even without data from psychological studies, there is no good reason to be hard on yourself. Your body does its best to be healthy and happy. It really does. It is in a constant state of regeneration and repair—it is a repairing powerhouse. The immune system, hormones, liver, lymph system, the very fabric of your DNA and cells...these are just some of the systems that are continually engaged in attempts to keep you as healthy as possible. Your body is always looking for ways to heal itself. Problems enter the picture when you do not trust these systems. If you do not trust your body and yourself, then you will begin to fear your body (if you do not fear it already). Fear makes war. Fear makes struggle. Fear makes punishment.

Without fear, however, you have the power to trust your body, to focus on the future, to have hope, and to heal. Fear calls for discipline and punishment. Love, on the other hand, calls for acceptance and forgiveness.

Acceptance, forgiveness, and love

Entirely at the fault of the Standard American Diet and Game, everyone's body has incurred at least some damage. This damage may be slight or it may be drastic. It may include obesity, diabetes, autoimmune disease, and other big-time hitters. It may be debilitating. It may be deadly. On the other hand, it may be as simple as insomnia or a bit of weight gain. Or it could be an invisible problem such as inflammation or nutrient deficiency. It could be an infinite variety of things, and it is at least one of them for all of us.

All of who you are today, including your cravings, habits, self-doubt, and fear, is a result of having lived through your own unique challenges. You have always done your best. You have always worked with whatever knowledge you had at your disposal. Your body has also always done its best. For that reason, you absolutely *must* forgive it. In fact, there is nothing to forgive. Your body has always been trying to heal. It has just been hindered by bad rules and bad food.

It's time for all of us women to accept ourselves for who we are. This doesn't mean that we need to stagnate—absolutely not. We still must set goals and strive toward them. We still must aspire toward better health and love in our lives. But we have to *own* who we are. I am Stefani Ruper. I was born to two relatively healthy parents who dieted throughout their lives. I was a perfectionist, and I developed self-punishing behaviors, and I accrued damage from starving myself for a significant period of time. I lived through infertility, largely due to my own behavior, but also due to the poor nutritional advice that my parents and I followed, and now all this baggage weighs heavily on me.

What's in your baggage? Can you see it objectively as something that must be accepted and forgiven? Can you accept and forgive all the things that have brought you to where you are today? Can you love and embrace who you are, in your own skin, the same way you might embrace other people?

These are important questions, and Step 5 details how to develop positive answers to them. Let it stand as a brief introduction here, then, that acceptance, forgiveness, and love are possibly the most powerful tools available to you. When you accept the context you are in, then you are empowered to move forward with forgiveness. Progress might not be perfect. Your body may take some time to heal. Changing your habits may take much longer than healing your body. But you move forward with knowledge of and forgiveness for all the difficulties you may have encountered on your journey. You acknowledge that your baggage may be *heavy*, and that it can take a long time to lighten these loads. Sometimes we think we have unpacked big chunks of it all at once, but then we realize that we never really got rid of it. It's not your fault. These burdens are big. The only option is to pick up where you left off and keep going.

In this model, when you eat more than you would like, or when you eat foods you are not supposed to eat because they are unhealthy, you don't have to beat yourself up. In fact, I insist that you do the opposite. That's the best way to be healthy in both body and mind. The reason you ate those foods is that certain cravings, ideas, or insecurities wound themselves tightly around the fibers of your brain. That's okay. You haven't gotten over them yet. So you forgive the episode—it happened. And you move forward loving your body, loving yourself, and loving your healing above all other things. Life is a journey, and there's no rush to the destination.

Your body is a complex, beautiful, and powerful healing machine. It is capable of a nearly infinite variety of things. It gives you life. It gives you breath. It gives you dancing and singing and joy and laughter. It processes food and turns it into energy, and this energy enables you to perform every single action that you will take in your life. This is a beautiful thing, and the more you respect how powerful it is, the more you can learn to trust your body. Sure, it might have accrued some damage over time. Sure, it might not be perfect. But it has a hell of a lot more things *right* with it than *wrong* with it, and the more you believe that, the easier it becomes to be in loving partnership.

Nature Rule #3 makes you sexy because

it starts you down the road of fixing your relationship with your body. Acceptance, forgiveness, love, and patience for the journey are some of the most powerful tools available to you for maintaining a good relationship with yourself. Being in harmony with your body and yourself is the number one requirement for being healthy and sexy.

Old Rule #4:
Warfare

Throughout this book, I use the language of relationship. I paint the picture of your body being separate from your mind—something that's pretty easy to do in the English language. It's a useful tool for conveying ideas simply and easily. It also just sort of *feels* right—you *are* in a relationship with your physical self.

Yet this language is a bit of an illusion. While I do talk about the body as a separate entity, it isn't. Bodies and minds are intricately interwoven. This is demonstrated by how powerful the placebo effect is—a vast majority of healing comes from *thinking* that you are being cured—and also by how intimately physical health can impact your mental health. One example is magnesium sufficiency: if you have insufficient magnesium stores, then you inevitably become more stressed, worried, and anxious than you would naturally be.

The practices of discipline and control that I debunk in Old Rules #1, 2, and 3 are wrapped up in this idea of separation between body and self. When the mind is separate from the body, it is easy to feel distanced, alienated, and at war.

When we see ourselves as separate from our bodies, it is pretty easy to blame, hate, and distrust our bodies. It is pretty easy to think that we are smarter than them, too. I tried that for a long time. I thought I could outwit my body—I could force it to be thin and have hormonal balance at the same time. Truth is, I couldn't. My body knew what it needed. I didn't. My job, as I finally came to understand after years of war, wasn't to control it, but rather to develop my understanding of those needs and then do my best to meet them. When my body and I were no longer at war, and I was no longer entrenched in a battle for control, we were liberated to move forward toward health together.

Nature Rule #4:
Harmony

You are at home no place in the universe the way you are in your body. In today's culture, we forget that. We don't treat our bodies like homes that we love. We treat them like enemies.

Nature teaches us, on the other hand, that we are one with our bodies. You *are* your body, whether you like it or not. There is no way around the fact that as a physical organism you have a complex, intimate, and unified relationship with your body.

Acknowledging how intimately tied you are to your body opens up a world of beautiful possibilities. Instead of seeing your body as a distinct entity that you need to control, your body can be your partner. You are not an alien in your body, but at home. You are not at war, but in an alliance. You do not control or restrict; you respect and you listen.

Bodies are powerful and beautiful things. Shouldn't we want to be at harmony with them? Shouldn't we want to have good relationships with them? Shouldn't it be a delight to treat them well so that they treat us well in return?

Nature Rule #4 makes you sexy because

it puts you at home in your skin. It helps you love and appreciate your body all the more, and be an *embodied* woman. The more embodied you are, the more you can feel at home in your physical self, and the more you can unapologetically and proudly be you.

Old Rule #5:
Bandages

Genetics are the scapegoat of our generation. When things go wrong, it's easy to say, "Well, that's just how it is," and leave it at that. The more we explore the human genome, the easier it is to sit back, blame our genes, and write off problems such as obesity and diabetes as inevitable. But we haven't learned everything yet. In fact, the more we learn about the genome, the more we realize that the story is more complicated. Remember the age-old debate of nature versus nurture? It turns out that nurture has never received its fair shake. It is *not* just nature that determines how healthy we are. Our genes *predispose* us to certain conditions, but the environment in which we live and the different conditions to which we expose our genes determine whether those disease triggers ever get tripped.

Nevertheless, society hasn't yet attained this level of wisdom. The Western world is still stuck on the idea of genetics. When we experience certain symptoms or develop certain disorders, we tend not to investigate the causes or think about the underlying conditions. We don't wonder why this problem happened in the first place or whether there is something we can do to fix it. Instead, we look to pharmaceuticals for easy solutions. Drugs are where we find the path of least resistance.

Bandages are a good metaphor for what's really going on in your body when you take drugs. When wounded, the body works hard to heal itself from the inside out. It is good at this. Sure, a bandage covers up the wound and prevents worse things from happening to it. But the bandage doesn't do any healing. The same goes

Bandages do not heal you. *You* heal you. for drugs. Drugs might cover up symptoms and make you feel better in the short term, but they rarely heal the underlying condition. Bandages do not heal you. *You* heal you.

In the case of scrapes and bruises, most people understand that the body is healing itself underneath the bandage. Yet when making decisions about more complex cases, such as heart disease, common sense goes out the window. Just about everyone involved forgets that the body is the only thing that can fix itself. No one seems to care that something went wrong for a *reason*. Nor do people seem to care all that much that there is a way to fix it. Doctors don't get it. Individuals don't get it. Pharmaceutical companies sure as hell don't get it. Instead, people often look to be saved by SSRIs, hormone replacement therapy, gene replacement therapy, antibiotics, or other medical interventions.

Simple examples demonstrate how we let ourselves slip in this regard. When most of us feel nauseated, we think: "What did I have for dinner last night?" There is a clear, easy-to-understand, cause-and-effect relationship between spoiled food and nausea. If you ate seafood that went bad, then you have an answer for your discomfort. Similarly, most people who get migraines learn over time what triggers them, whether it is bright lights, loud sounds, stress, or certain foods. And when we feel wide awake and then crash into exhausted oblivion, we have a pretty good hunch that it's because of the cupcake we ate with lunch.

In all these cases, cause-and-effect reasoning explains what happened. A certain stimulus or behavior had a certain effect, as both science and common sense made clear. Understanding this relationship provides a means to figure out how to avoid that ailment the next time. The same goes for diabetes, obesity, heart disease, cancer, and so many other health problems. Just because they are more complicated does not mean that they do not have their own sets of causes. The trick is to figure out what those causes are and then to make the diet and lifestyle changes necessary to reverse them.

Drugs can be appropriate

Of course, there are many instances in which drugs and other medical interventions are helpful. For one thing, given the amount of damage that the Standard American Diet has already done to our bodies, some symptoms or diseases are beyond overcoming with food.

For example, Hashimoto's thyroiditis is an autoimmune disease that attacks the thyroid gland. While a woman with Hashimoto's might regain some natural thyroid function once she fixes her diet, some of her thyroid gland may have been damaged beyond repair, so she'll need to take thyroid hormone in the form of supplements for optimal health.

Another example is radiation or chemotherapy. If I get any type of cancer, I am going to use whatever resources I need—inclusive of diet and drugs—in order to heal.

Additionally, it may be appropriate or desirable to manage symptoms while making diet and lifestyle changes. Smart intervention can speed healing. The point here is that drugs cannot replace healing. They must be secondary. Otherwise, true, lifelong health will forever be out of reach.

Nature Rule #5:
Healing

Today's most advanced science tells us that the story of genetics is not necessarily the right one. Genes certainly play a role in what sorts of traits and illnesses crop up in a person's life, but they are only part of the story. Just as important as genes, if not more so, is the environment in which the genes are situated. No gene will leap into action without being provoked. For example, you will not become overweight—even if your genes predispose you to do so—unless you eat the kinds of foods and do the kinds of things that flick the genes' "on" switch.

Things go wrong for a reason. They go wrong as a result of being forced to interact with elements for which the body was not built. Examples abound: cubicles, jetlag, and fluorescent lights are as important as Snickers bars, French fries, and soda. I am not spouting New Age idealism here. This is real, hard science. Unnatural foods, chemicals, and behaviors send the body into panic mode: it simply does not know how to handle them. It wasn't built for them. What is it supposed to do with chemicals made in a laboratory—chemicals it has never seen before in the whole of human history?

One example is trans fats. The body has no need for them and no reason for or means by which to handle them. Trans fats are completely new and unfamiliar chemicals. They're so unfamiliar that the body straight up does not know what to do with them. It's no wonder that consuming them derails normal, healthy metabolism, perhaps permanently.

Other examples of unhealthy, unnatural foods abound. Processed sugar is one. Omega-6 seed oils are another. Proteins in grain products turn whole grains into potential threats.

The thing is, our bodies do their best to heal and to be healthy. They are naturally healthy. But how can they do their jobs when we regularly flood them with chemicals that interrupt and even destroy normal processes? Across the Western world, millions of unhealthy and overweight people have demonstrated over and over again that aligning their diets and lifestyles with what their bodies were designed for melts off fat, lowers disease risk, clears skin, and provides greater energy. Natural food gives the body all the tools it needs to make its own repairs. Nothing in the world is a more powerful medicine than giving your body the building blocks it is constantly, desperately crying out for.

More evidence that confirms this hypothesis can be found in the animal kingdom. Is cancer, heart disease, or obesity found in the wild? No. Are there autoimmune conditions? No. Crooked teeth or cavities? No. Acne? No. What about in the zoo? Yeah, sometimes there is disease there. But why? That's an easy answer. When animals are removed from their natural habitats, they often become sick. They might even refuse to reproduce, as pandas sometimes do. The same goes for pets. Some pets today get very sick. But dogs and cats never used to become ill, and dogs and cats in the wild do not have the same problems as the ones to which we give dog or cat food. Dog food companies have noticed this issue and have begun developing lines of food specifically built for dogs' needs. Grain-free, corn-free, and sugar-free dog foods now line store shelves. If we can understand that dogs, cats, and animals in the zoo fare better with natural diets, then shouldn't it be the same for us?

The same even goes for plants. We all understand that plants have different water needs. The daisies in my yard need to be watered every couple of days, but if I water my cactus, it shrivels up within hours. The same thing applies to us. If I overeat something unhealthy, or if I undereat something I need, I am going to shrivel up within hours. My dog, cat, and panda will all do the same.

This is the basic fact that grounds the *Sexy by Nature* Golden Rule in science. The human body is built for specific foods. All bodies are. When it is deprived of these foods and fed other things instead, it gets sick. Diseases such as cancer, heart disease, Alzheimer's, diabetes, obesity, and autoimmune diseases are found only in societies that consume high levels of industrialized foods, such as America. As a matter of fact, as cultures all over the world industrialized and began to consume processed foods, researchers documented the rise of disease over time.

The *Sexy by Nature* Golden Rule Reminder: *Your body is a natural body with natural needs that, when loved properly, loves you right back.*

Nature Rule #5 is actually one of the most empowering. It shows us the way forward. It teaches us how to heal ourselves. It shows us what we need to do to prevent and overcome ailments. We are not doomed. Genes do not make us sick; bad foods and bad behavior do. This fact might scare you—it gives you a lot of responsibility—but it shouldn't. It's easy to nourish yourself. I will show you how. Health and lifelong sexiness are at your fingertips.

Nature Rule #5 makes you sexy because

it enables you to achieve Health with a capital H. With this rule, you do not have to rely on drugs to cover up your symptoms. You are not tricked by the conventional idea that disease is inevitable and that you are powerless to prevent or fight it. You are empowered with scientific knowledge of what human bodies need. You are empowered with a loving and respectful relationship with your body. And you have the tools you need to move forward toward greater healing, health, and sex appeal.

Old Rule #6:
Unquestioning ignorance

Health would be easy if all the industries out there had our best interests at heart. It would be even easier if government and news agencies understood health. Unfortunately, neither of those scenarios is true. The supermarket is a dizzying array of products clamoring for your attention and addiction. Nutrition labels are confusing. The government's dietary advice falls depressingly short of the pace of cutting-edge science. It's not just impossible to know what to eat these days; it is also impossible to know whom to listen to about what to eat.

I do my best to navigate all this confusion in our culture, and I take advice and make positive choices where I can. In my past life, this meant that I turned to the government's food recommendations, to health claims on food labels, and to what I heard about or read on the Internet. This would have been a good thing if it weren't for the fact that I was systematically misled on a regular basis. No one was out to hurt me intentionally (most likely), but due to a wide variety of blunders and mishaps, the government, the pharmaceutical industry, and popular culture do not do health right. It wasn't until I acquired the skills to question them (Nature Rule #6) that I could move beyond them and make real change for long-term health.

The government and food

As nice as it would be for food recommendations to be objective, that's a bit of a pipe dream. They are impossibly tied up with money, lobbies, and bureaucracy, and that's not going to change anytime soon.

The federal government updates its dietary guidelines every five years. The much-anticipated, most recent recommendations were revealed in 2010. The revolutionary new spin on things? The USDA now recommends a food plate rather than a pyramid.

The plate is a genuine step up from the pyramid in a handful of ways. First, recommendations changed from an explicit number of servings to proportions, allowing people of all sizes to follow the guidelines. As a 5′2″ woman, for example, I am no longer advised to eat an egregious eleven servings of grain each day. Instead, I am now advised to make grains 20 percent of my total food intake. The fact that the old pyramid recommended *eleven servings* of whole grains is a problem in and of itself. Grains are a nutritionally empty food. At 20 percent, MyPlate has reduced the grain recommendation somewhat. It has also divided the rest of a healthy diet among vegetables, fruits, protein, and dairy. That's not horrible advice.

But the plate still fails in one very big way: it does not account for the quality of the foods being consumed. It technically does not distinguish between French fries and carrot sticks as vegetables, for example. MyPlate gives me free rein to eat (and public school lunch programs to sell) as many French fries as I want and pretend that it's healthy.

Worse, these recommendations are made under the influence of food lobbies. The meat, egg, and dairy lobbies are well known for how much sway they hold in Washington. Less often demonized but perhaps even more powerful are the wheat, corn, and soy industries. The government's advice is dictated at least in part by which industry has the most gold in its pockets and by how important it is to sell food for the economy to grow.

Moreover, the genuine good efforts of people such as First Lady Michelle Obama and others on the side of government are inevitably stunted by how poor nutritional science in the government is. What if the government doesn't understand health? (Because it doesn't.) What if government food standards are behind the times in terms of nutritional science? (Because they are.) What if all the nutritionists in the United States were required to agree with the federal government on what is healthy? (Because they are.) All these things are true. Worse, however, is the incredible inertia of government and public processes. Well-intentioned health advocates are woefully behind in terms of the quality of health science, largely due to the simple fact of red tape. If we listen to the government in pursuit of good health, we inevitably fail.

The food industry and food

The American people were a fit and healthy group of vibrant women and men until the latter half of the 20th century. BMIs were in healthy ranges. Cancer wasn't an issue. Diabetes was a disease that attacked only the very old. Skin was relatively clear. Senior citizens were relatively active and mentally well.

The best part? No one really had to try. In the good old days, health (provided a certain socioeconomic status) was a bit of a given. Breakfast, lunch, and dinner were prepared at home, and the whole family sat down to eat together. Foods—even the questionably canned and Frankenstein forms of the 1950s—were relatively natural compared to the foods we eat today. Preservatives were only just beginning to leak into the American diet. Spam was too new to have damaged anyone beyond repair. Soda was still a treat and was lower in sugar than it is today.

In 1960, weight was relatively stable in America. Women ages 20–29 averaged about 128 pounds. By 2000, however, the average weight of that group had reached 157. In that forty-year period, weight increased across all ages and groups. Adults, teenagers, and children were heavier. And every age group was heavier than the one preceding it—indicating that people were gaining weight throughout their lives.[5]

What had crept in over time was the food *industry*. Before the 20th century, food was grown on farms and eaten. Makes sense to me! But by the end of the 20th century, food had become something that was *made*. It was *prepared. Served*. A marketable commodity. Food was no longer sustenance from the home—it was convenient, flashy, addictive, hip. It was an advertiser's dream.

> The American diet has exploded into a highly palatable, highly convenient, nearly-impossible-to-resist orgy of flavor and texture, and we can hardly be blamed for eating it.

The result has been drastic increases in the consumption of deep-fried fats, sugar, and processed foods. Almost no one shops solely in the produce aisle these days. Produce used to be the only thing sold in markets. Now, the produce aisle is one of approximately twelve, with entire aisles devoted to soda, fruit juices, condiments, breakfast cereals, baking goods, frozen dinners, meal replacements, candy, packaged desserts, chips, pretzels, and diet foods. If you want an answer for what has happened to the American diet, it is this: it has exploded into a highly palatable, highly convenient, nearly-impossible-to-resist orgy of flavor and texture, and we can hardly be blamed for eating it. We can hardly be blamed at all.

Foods are explicitly designed to be addictive. The more you crave them, the more you eat. The more you eat, the more you buy. The more you buy, the more others profit. These simple equations have the power to destroy lives. The food industry has a vested interest in keeping you coming back for more. Many food companies will do nearly anything to promote consumption, whether it's taste-testing a soda for the right amount of addictive flavors for years before it is "perfected" and deemed suitable for release to the public, designing cereal boxes with irresistibly charming leprechauns on them, or developing "healthy" alternatives that trick us into thinking we are doing the right thing by buying them.

This last point is particularly scary. What happens when someone with a vested interest in selling a product starts playing with sneaky ways to justify slapping a "healthy" label on it?

There are infinite examples of how most (though not all) health claims made by the food industry are bogus. The supermarket is full of them.

One example that demonstrates the depth of this problem is omega-3 peanut butter. What's the issue? Peanut butter is composed primarily of omega-6 fat. This is not a good thing for the peanut butter industry because eating too much omega-6 fat relative to omega-3 fat is unhealthy, and people have begun to catch on to this fact. In response, the industry has created a peanut product that is more "balanced." One company calls this new peanut product Smart Balance—something that is supposed to be healthy for you. Further inspection reveals, however, that far less omega-3 is added to the peanut butter than would be required for a significantly healthy balance. I have seen peanut butters that have as little as 0.2 grams of omega-3 fat compared to 6 grams of omega-6. That's still a ratio of 1:30—not unlike saying that 30 glasses of wine is a nice balance to one night's dinner. This is where the advertising is deceptive. It claims that something is healthy. I suppose it is health*ier*—but it is not nearly the miracle the label leads us to believe.

Moreover, most peanut butters use flaxseed as the source of omega-3 fatty acids. (This is true of the Smart Balance variety.) The problem is that the only kinds of omega-3 fat that have the power to balance omega-6 are EPA and DHA fats, and they are found in high quantities only in seafood. The kind of omega-3 found in flaxseed is ALA. The body can convert ALA into EPA and DHA, but at a conversion rate so low that your immune system would never know the difference. For this reason, the "smart balancing act" that this peanut butter product claims to do does not really happen at all.

Who is to blame for this poor mimicry of "healthy"? The food industry? Perhaps. Perhaps it knows that this is the real story, and perhaps it is aware of its deceptions. In some instances of this kind of "healthy" advertising, I am sure that this is the case. But it is also possible that these companies do not have a good grip on the detailed science. Either of the two options is unsatisfactory: the food industry is either deceptive or poorly educated. This is one of the primary reasons to avoid processed foods, period. Why experiment with designed foods? Why mess around with the unnatural formulas of processed foods when natural foods are plentiful?

* * *

Even more simple and scary examples abound. Diet soda may be worse for us than the real stuff, depending on how future studies pan out. Breakfast cereals are fortified with vitamins and minerals that are poorly absorbed by the body in fortified form, and that—as in the case of folic acid—have been linked to different cancers. "No high-fructose corn syrup" does not really mean that a food is all that much better for you; it means only that it contains a different kind of sugar. And when a candy bar claims that it's a rich source of protein because it's got 4 grams of peanuts squeezed in among 250 calories of chemicals, food dyes, sugar, and trans fats, someone from the company that manufactures it should be kicked in the shins. Hard.

We find ourselves duped in this way day in and day out. It's not our fault. In my quest for good health, before I turned to natural foods, I took advice where I heard and read it. When a label said that a product was a smart balance between omega-3 and omega-6 fats, well, sign me up, I'd say! Since then, I have learned to default to skepticism. I read every nutrition label with a raised eyebrow, and more often than not I cringe or roll my eyes before placing the item carefully back on the shelf.

It's nearly impossible to navigate the landscape. Nonetheless, we know that taking the food industry's and even the government's word for it is not the way to find good health. For that, we must turn to science, nature, and our own rigorous common sense.

Nature Rule #6:
Investigation

Opposed to popular culture, the food industry, and poor governmental advice, there are excellent methods for figuring out which foods we should eat. Questioning authority, investigating on our own, using our own experience and common sense, and learning from the diets and habits of existing hunter-gatherer and traditional populations are all crucial investigative tools that are radically underutilized by mainstream nutritionism. My personal success, and the success that millions of people around the world on similar diets, has convinced me that the *Sexy by Nature* diet promotes the best and fastest healing.

Good science

In some ways it is easy to distinguish "good" science from "bad," and in other ways it is very difficult. It's easy because once you've gotten the hang of it, you can smell bad science from a mile away. Bad science includes exclamation points, sweeping generalizations, egregious statements of cause and effect (such as "eggs cause heart disease"; the better statement would be "eggs contain dietary cholesterol"), overarching statements, and false premises, such as starting off with the idea that pharmaceuticals are the best way to treat a problem. Good science, on the other hand, acknowledges its limitations, does its best to account for all variables, never asserts a cause unless it is obvious, and steps carefully around other theories. Bad science is sensationalist. Bad science makes headlines. Bad science is often popular. Good science is thorough. Good science uses all the data. Good science often goes unnoticed, overshadowed by the exultant claims of medical gurus with TV shows who get paid to endorse products.

It can still be challenging to discern the difference between good and bad science sometimes. In these cases significant scientific training and rigorous analysis are required. Not all of us have time for this, so we either have to find analysts we trust or use other methods for knowing. I honestly believe that I am an analyst you can trust. There are people with even greater levels of specialization and expertise on whom I rely.

Existing hunter-gatherer and traditional populations

One thing that can be said with absolute certainty about the Western diet is that it messes people up. Time and time again, native populations around the globe have encountered the sweets, grains, and unnatural foods of the Western diet and watched their waistlines balloon, their skin become pockmarked, and their death rates run high off a cliff. This is far from a laughing matter, and everyone knows it: the Western diet deranges health, often precipitously.

As far as we can tell, no extant hunter-gatherer or foraging cultures (of which there are at least a few) who eat their natural diets have more than the tiniest incidence of obesity, skin conditions, crooked teeth, osteoporosis, heart disease, cancer, diabetes, or any of the wide class of autoimmune diseases. These natural diets may be largely fish based, as in the Inuit population, game and vegetable based, as in many Native American traditional cultures, or composed of starches, pork, fowl, coconut, seafood, and fish, as is the case with many Pacific Island populations such as the Kitavans and Hawaiian Islanders. Consider the Okinawans, renowned centenarians, whose diet consists largely of pork products, lard, white rice, sweet potatoes, eggs, fish, seaweed, and other vegetables. Diets vary widely across the globe. Yet what do all of them have in common? No preservatives. No chemicals. No processed foods. No grains. No sugar. No deep fryers.

From these facts, we can infer that America's current diet is no small player in the health crisis. The human body is programmed for its natural environment—how could it not be?—and as far as we can tell from looking at these cultures, they are made up of lithe, strong, powerful, long-lived, shiny-toothed, and beautiful human beings.

I do not mean to idealize these cultures and individuals. Human beings are simply human beings. But there is a quality to foraging health that the Western body lacks. These people live and act as natural beings, and they eat only natural foods. Their diets span a huge variety, but they are all *natural* and therefore coherent with what the human body has evolved to eat.

Comparing our diets and lifestyle habits to those of existing hunter-gatherer cultures is a great way to learn about what is healthy and what isn't. It shows us ways in which we may be doing it incorrectly and can help us determine what our paths forward should look like.

Listening

Living organisms are wired to work intuitively. Consider a dog, a gorilla, or even a human baby, for example. They know when to start eating and when to stop. They know when to sleep and when to wake. They don't need to be told. They don't need to be controlled. Instead, they do these things intuitively.

Today, we often hear and say that we need to listen to our bodies. Listening is a common trope that floats under the currents of our cultural norms. I say it, too, and I mean it profoundly. *Nothing* in the world is more powerful for healing than letting the body speak and letting its needs be your top priority.

What I mean when I say "listen," however, is a bit more nuanced than what others might mean.

The problem is that we are bombarded with foods, advertisements, and enticements that make it hard to discern a natural bodily signal from a signal that's been hijacked. Refined sugar is addictive, for example. Therefore, listening to your body's craving for lollipops might not be the best way to achieve true health. Your desires and needs are regularly hijacked by the Standard American Diet and Game. It's almost impossible to resist in such a rabidly consumer-driven and fast-paced world.

So how do you listen to your body?

First, you eliminate the things from your diet that hijack your senses. Or at least you do your best to educate yourself about them and navigate them as safely, cautiously, and lovingly as possible. This means that you stop driving past that fast-food restaurant that smells *so good*. It means that you cut sugar out of your diet and stop it from sending your body on a blood sugar roller coaster. And it means that you teach yourself about the toxins inherent in the foods constantly being marketed to you (by doing things like reading this book!). Over time, you will stop desiring these foods because your senses will come back under your own control. The more you value your health, too, the less appealing these foods will become. Why eat something that is going to poison you and make you overweight? In the end, it stops being worth it.

Once you eliminate the hijackers, you have the glorious freedom to listen without doubting yourself. Within the range of natural foods and in a natural lifestyle, the body's hormones work the way they are supposed to. You crave the right foods. You sleep when you need to. You exercise when you need to.

Without sense hijackers, you naturally, effortlessly, and seamlessly give your body exactly what it needs. It becomes as natural to you as it does to other animals in the kingdom. You don't have to fight. You just have to listen. Sometimes it's difficult to get to this place. I understand that, and I discuss how to do so in greater depth in later chapters.

Hardcore common sense

The last but most important method you should use to figure out what your body needs is hardcore common sense. This relates very much to the point above. Yes, listening is important. More important, however, is that the signals you hear need to come through a filter of common sense. Where is my craving for Cheerios coming from? Is that a natural need or an emotional attachment? Chances are good that it's an emotional attachment, and loyalty to common sense will save the day.

Hardcore common sense also helps us discern what is good versus what is bad, whom we should trust, and how we want to approach eating. For example, there's no way I can prove to you with 100 percent certainty that the *Sexy by Nature* way of living and eating is the right way. There are hundreds of competing schools and ideas out there. But your hardcore common sense will tell you what makes the most sense to you. Does it make more sense to be at war with your body or to work with it? Does it make more sense to heal your body from the get-go or to try to bandage it up later? Does it make more sense to think of your body as a natural body or as a thing that is distant from you and requires medication? Does it make more sense to care about the quantity of calories or the quality of calories? For each of these questions, I share with you my opinion. And if my opinion makes sense to you based on your experience and observation and makes its way through your filters of common sense, then it is worth a shot. It might be the best shot you take for your body in your whole life.

Nature Rule #6 makes you sexy because

it gives you a better idea of what you should be eating. It gives you the tools you need to make smart decisions. It empowers you and makes you the boss of your own life. It puts your healing and your health in your own sexy, capable hands. It heals you and transforms you. It also facilitates harmony with your body because it asks you to listen to your body and do your best to meet its needs.

Old Rule #7:
Sexism

Let's be honest: men's bodies can tolerate a lot more crap than women's can. Men can fast all day without repercussions. They can lose all the weight they want (and quickly!) without hurting themselves. They can eat very-low-carbohydrate diets. They can exercise day in and day out without getting acne or becoming insomniacs. Of course, it is possible for these things to happen to men, but they happen at a much lower rate. (It's also possible for them *not* to happen to women. These issues are just much more common in women.) Men's bodies have none of the delicate machinery that the reproductive system laces throughout the female body, and therefore none of the special concerns.

As far as I can tell, very few people in the diet world pay attention to the fact that the female body has distinct needs. These needs mean that health and weight loss must be understood from a female perspective in order to be done in the healthiest and most efficient ways possible. Yet they simply are not, and women's lives are made worse for it every day. Women's bodies are more sensitive to the negative effects of psychological stress. Hormones are easily upset by starvation (which the body senses when calories are severely restricted). Weight loss for women stalls much more easily than it does for men. Thyroid function often shuts down in response to starvation signals and poor nutrient status.

Worse is that women experience dozens of health problems at rates twice that or more of men—and still we receive little special attention. More women have acne than men. More women report experiencing anxiety and depression. More women are insomniacs. Women also deal with a host of problems that men never have to. PMS, PMDD, endometriosis, adenomyosis, cysts, fibroids, thyroid disorders, and polycystic ovarian syndrome are just a few of the conditions that demand attention and deserve respect, but that fly under the radar simply because they are female.

Nature Rule #7:
Female empowerment

The final smart rule from nature is that the female body is a distinct body with different needs than a man's. Having a solid understanding of the female body enables us to develop weight-loss and health goals specifically targeted at and optimized for women. The more we appreciate the unique aspects of the female body, the better our approach to it, and therefore our lives, will be.

What is a female body?

A female body is distinct from a male body because of its reproductive function. It is capable of incredible power—building an entire organism within itself and of itself!—and then birthing, nursing, and raising that little baby. It can even do this multiple times, a miracle built upon miracles if I've ever heard of one.

This great power comes at a great price, or perhaps with great responsibility. A better way to look at it might be that this great gift requires specific nurturing. The female body doesn't take crap from anybody or anything. It won't have its babies messed with. For this reason, it can shut down reproductive function at the slightest drop of a nutritional hat. This is bad if you want to make babies. It is also bad if hormone balance is one of your priorities, as it should be. Hormone balance is responsible for good mental health, clear skin, and fat burning, among other things. Healthy hormones make for a healthy woman, so we had best listen to what our hormones want from us.

There are two predominant ways in which dysregulation occurs. One is excess, and the other is restriction. Excess is a problem because being overweight and diseased is a burden that the body does not handle very well. The hormone condition polycystic ovarian syndrome, for example, which causes infertility, is largely correlated with insulin resistance and being overweight and affects roughly 15 percent of women.[6] Excess is a stressor, and it shows.

Restriction is a problem because it tells the body that famine is looming and it's not a good time to make a baby. Dieting, low-calorie eating, fasting, excess exercise, rapid weight loss, low levels of body fat, and, perhaps worst of all, psychological stress make the body feel starved and therefore put a halt to reproductive function.

Symptoms of hormone imbalance occur on both ends of the spectrum. Poor skin quality, acne, fatigue, anxiety, depression, insomnia, low libido, difficulty with weight maintenance, PMS, menstrual cramps, and male-pattern hair growth are all realities that women's bodies fight against every day.

What does a woman's body need?

The female body needs to be treated as a natural body to which these sorts of things can happen. It is not a machine that can be hacked with medicine. It may get by on these perspectives for some time, but it will never heal by them, nor will it find true, radiant health without side effects.

When left to its own devices, a woman's body is a natural thing that takes care of its natural needs on its own. It will ovulate when it thinks it has the resources available to ovulate, and it won't if it doesn't. It also does other kinds of healing on its own: it heals itself of pathogens and viruses; it keeps hormones in proper balance; and it maintains proper hunger signals in order to promote healthy weight maintenance.

The female body has the know-how and the capability to make itself strong, functioning, energetic, and radiant. Bodies are not meant to be broken. They are not meant to be sick and tired and pockmarked. They are meant to be excited, healthy, and joyful. All you have to do to make that happen is to give your body the fuel it is designed to run on. It will do all the heavy lifting itself.

Nature Rule #7 makes you sexy because

it provides you with the knowledge you need to develop an intimate relationship with your body. The more you know about yourself, the healthier you can be. The more you understand your health and weight-loss needs, the more you can live into, take advantage of, and love your femininity. The more you appreciate how different and special the female body is, the more excited you can be to be in the skin you're in.

The Takeaway:
Out with the old and in with the new

Seven old rules to do away with, and seven good ones to take their place. Seven concepts that prevent good health, and seven that lead to empowered, embodied, and healthy natural womanhood. Seven problems, and seven solutions.

The gist of the new rules is this:

The best way to achieve health, sex appeal, and happiness is to work *with* rather than *over* or *against* the body. It is to start from square one in terms of how we understand our bodies, and to appreciate their true nature and power. It is to understand that things happen to our bodies for a reason, and that we can influence those events by feeding our bodies better food, giving them better nourishment, and providing them with the support they need in order to heal. Nature is the real name of the game. Nature tells us the real essence of our bodies. Nature provides us with the means we need to heal. Nature gives us the health, vibrancy, and harmony with our bodies that we need in order to be not just fine, but excellent.

Nature. Harmony. Love. Empowerment. These are the new rules that change the rules. I call this step "Trailblaze" because it does exactly that. It is new. Radical. Radically *easy*. This is not the old game. It is not the struggle that everyone else is entrenched in. Real health is not a battle. It is an alliance. It's peace. It's listening and nurturing and harmony. It's setting forth on new ground with natural principles that have the power to rock the feminine world.

2: Nourish

The best way to transform a body into a sexy body is to build it out of the right stuff.

Think about this in terms of building a house. A house must be built out of something—straw, sticks, or bricks. In the exact same way, your body must be made out of something—and that something is the food you eat. Scientists have analyzed samples and have concluded that American skin and hair is about 67 percent corn.[7]

You have the option to build your house out of the wrong stuff (like corn). Since the foundational materials would be so weak, you'd have to spend an inordinate amount of your time doing repairs: spending hours each day at the gym, for example, or relying on drugs and taking supplements. An alternative would be to max out your credit cards in an effort to disguise your body's "walls" with clothes, makeup, and cosmetic surgery—doing your best to distract everyone around you from the fact that your house is crumbling.

The other option is to build your house out of the right stuff. Just as the strongest, sturdiest house is made from the best materials, so the strongest, sexiest bodies are made from the best materials. Instead of poorly supported straw, your house should be built out of bricks and mortar. This will protect you from decades of Big Bad Wolf attacks.

Natural versus "Natural" Foods

The vast majority of experts agree that the healthiest foods are the most natural ones. For this reason, most health gurus advocate a diet based on natural foods. Michael Pollan is a prominent example. Dean Ornish, Mehmet Oz, Mark Bittman, Jonathan Safran Foer, and T. Colin Campbell are other big-name players on that list. Moreover, I bet that nearly every American who eats fast food, snacks on chips, guzzles soda, or lives off of Slurpees would admit that they don't think their diets are all that healthy. Processed foods are bad, and everyone knows this quite well.

If you asked Pollan, Ornish, Oz, and everyone else I mentioned what the most natural and healthful foods are, you'd end up with a long and diverse list. Some would say soy is the best food on the planet, whereas I think soy is one of the worst. Some love bacon, and others think it's the plague. Some are militant vegans who are committed to forgoing all animal products, and others are militant omnivores, insisting that animal products are a healthy part of a balanced diet. Some think bread should be a staple of the American diet, while others (myself included) think that bread verges on poisonous.

The problem is that we all define "natural" differently.

* * *

Sexy by Nature is founded largely on the idea that most people's ideas about "natural" are wrong. Why? Because they fail to use the principles of investigation I laid out earlier of good science, attention to existing hunter-gatherer populations, and common sense.

The hunter-gatherer principle is what makes my views different from those of most health advocates. Few of the health advocates listed above have ever investigated, let alone written about, the diets of people who still live naturally off the land. I and many smart people on whom I rely have. For this reason, Pollan, Bittman, Oz, and others' recommendations fall woefully short of the apparent magical properties of truly natural diets (and diets that attempt to approximate them, such as the one I recommend in this book). Sure, these advocates forbid sugar, trans fats, and processing chemicals, which are all very important to avoid. But what about other foods that no extant hunter-gatherer cultures eat, such as grains like bread, omega-6 oils like vegetable oil, and estrogenic foods like soy? These foods are abundant on the often-recommended Mediterranean Diet, though studies have indicated that a more traditional diet that eliminates them, such as the *Sexy by Nature* diet, is a superior method for treating type 2 diabetes.[8] Going the extra mile—or finishing the *first* mile in the first place—in terms of what is "natural" transforms what would otherwise be a ho-hum approach to nutrition into a potent supply of the glory and radiance of natural womanhood.

Almost no obesity, tooth decay, diabetes, or other noncommunicable diseases beset traditional populations such as the Inuit, Kitavans, and !Kung Bushmen. These people are typically vibrant, athletic, and strong, with the clearest skin and straightest teeth I have ever seen. The diet I describe here couples the best science that has been unearthed on foods to date with wisdom garnered from nature and the people who still live in nature. It is, in fact, founded on the exact same principles as Paleo diets, primal diets, and the like. What these approaches to health all have in common is that they tirelessly pursue the question of what it means to be human and how best to live as natural beings, and I would be amiss to forgo mentioning what a great debt *Sexy by Nature* owes to the brilliance of researchers and advocates in the Paleolithic realm. Being one of these diets that pursue the right natural foods for natural bodies, *Sexy by Nature* leads to profound harmony. It makes for serious healing. And it empowers you to build your house out of the absolute best materials on the planet.

Other "natural" health advocates and I agree that...

Natural foods cannot be found in the aisles of grocery stores. They are not found in bags or boxes.

This principle rules out anything that contains processing chemicals or preservatives and almost everything that contains more than a few ingredients. None of the processing chemicals that scientists have recently invented are suited for or recognizable to the human body. They are foreign agents, and the body doesn't know how to handle them.

When you eat foods that your body doesn't recognize, it panics. Try as it might to heal itself and be healthy, it cannot succeed if harmful foods constantly work against it. It doesn't matter if it's low-calorie, sugar-replaced, low-fat, or low-carbohydrate; no amount of chemical tweaking will make an unhealthy food healthy. If it has chemicals in it, it is quite likely not good for you.

Sexy by Nature says...

A truly natural food is one that can be found in the wild.

If you were dropped in the Rockies and left to survive on your own, what would you eat? If you were dropped in the savanna, what would you eat? If you were dropped on an island in the Pacific, what would you eat?

Natural foods have never been processed, milled, separated, or distilled to any significant degree in factories. Most health advocates fail to account for this. Which foods are accepted by gurus but fail this test? Seed oils, including canola oil, vegetable oil, soybean oil, and corn oil. Processed dairy products. Cereal. Bread. Anything labeled low-fat.

Foods that can be found in the wild are the ones humans have consumed for two million years. These are the best foods to eat because over the course of history the human body became well equipped to eat them. Other potentially healthful options have

slipped into the human diet in the last several thousand years—
the body does have the ability to adapt quickly. But if a food was
introduced to humans in the last several thousand years—a fright-
eningly short period when compared to the whole two million years
of human evolution—or especially if it was introduced in the last
few decades, there's a good chance that it is not an optimal food.

More on vegetarianism

Many natural health advocates still play by the old rules,
particularly by adhering to the principles of vegetarianism. They
insist that vegetarianism is the healthiest diet, and they attempt
to back up this claim with studies comparing the health of
vegetarians to non-vegetarians. One of the primary legs on which
this argument stands is inherently flawed, however. Statistics
have shown many times over that vegetarians have a lower risk
of heart disease and other noncommunicable diseases relative to
non-vegetarians. This would be all well and good if it weren't for
the fact that vegetarians are also the most educated, the most
health-conscious, the most athletic, and the least likely to smoke,
do drugs, or drink alcohol. When these other factors are taken into
account, vegetarianism stops appearing to indicate superior health.

It has also been argued that a vegetarian or vegan diet is the
natural human diet. This hypothesis has been proved wrong on a
wide variety of fronts. For example:

- As I mentioned in Step 1, the human body requires vitamin
  B_{12}, a nutrient that comes only from animal products, in order
  to survive, as well as choline, DHA, heme iron, vitamin A, and
  other nutrients found primarily in meat.

- The human digestive track is too small and delicate for an
  entirely plant-based (and especially raw) diet.

- The body has significant protein needs that cannot be met in
  the wild without animal products.

- Human teeth are constructed for an omnivorous diet—one
  composed of both plant and animal foods.

What Makes a Food Healthy?

Every time you eat, you have the ability to hurt or heal your body. Ask yourself: Is this food not just full of nutrients but also built to be digested and assimilated? Is this food gentle on all the organs and full of loving nourishment rather than insidious threats?

A number of factors affect the nourishing potential of foods. An orange, for example, provides quick energy in the form of sugar with a heavy dose of vitamin C. A sirloin steak, on the other hand, provides slow-burning protein for cellular repair and function as well as a host of vitamins and minerals, such as iron, copper, zinc, vitamin B_6, and vitamin B_{12}.

More importantly, however, the foods you eat need to be happily, gently, and gratefully received by your body. It doesn't matter how much vitamin C a food has if it also contains 100 grams of high-fructose corn syrup that will disrupt your hunger and fat-storage mechanisms, or if it contains unnatural proteins that will damage your intestines. One example of this, of many, is "vitamin-enriched" breakfast cereal. What breakfast cereal enrichment adds in the way of vitamins is minimal compared to the damage it can do underneath.

Bad foods can show their ugly stripes in nearly infinite places in the body, but we can talk about them in a few big, important categories. The first is digestion. The digestive system is the one system explicitly designed to interact with food—it is your body's interface with the external world. After digestion we'll look at the immune system and metabolic hormones, both of which are also highly sensitive to your diet and play crucial roles in your overall health.

> ## Skimming
>
> Some of the explanations that follow may be too detailed or scientific for your tastes. In that case, more power to you! Skimming is fine, and the takeaway points at the end of each section should give you an adequate understanding for your goals.

Health interaction #1: your gut and its inhabitants

The digestive system is the gateway to the body. Everything that moves through your intestines is still in some sense *outside* of the body. It hasn't gotten in yet. So, when you eat a food, what happens to it? How does it get in? What regulates the process of absorption? One of the first steps is interacting with gut bacteria. Trillions of bacteria live in your gut and regulate the breakdown of food into nutrients. These bacteria are, in a sense, like castle guards. As foods march through your digestive track, these guards help keep order and promote healthy digestive processes.

The more and higher quality of gut bacteria you have, the healthier your kingdom is. The fewer of them you have, the less protection your digestive system has, and the more vulnerable the rest of your body is to damage and disrepair. Having a healthy gut flora population is crucial for maintaining good overall health.

Your gut flora is characterized by the type and amount of bacteria you have. The flora can be balanced toward good bacteria, which is a healthy situation, or toward bad bacteria, which is an unhealthy situation.

Gut flora:

A fancy term for gut bacteria. It might fascinate you to learn that there are more of these fellas in your body than your own cells. The bacteria in your gut number in the trillions, which is up to ten times the amount of human cells you have, and the mass of bacteria swimming in your gut clocks in at around 3 pounds. A large percentage of your stool is dead bacteria. You wouldn't be able to digest food or have bowel movements without gut bacteria.

Health benefits of good gut bacteria

Healthy gut bacteria perform a variety of important functions. Increasing healthy gut flora through diet or probiotic supplementation helps regulate blood sugar, improves insulin sensitivity, mitigates depression and other mental health disorders, minimizes inflammation and infection, promotes weight loss, and prevents allergies, asthma, and autoimmune disease. The reason gut bacteria can do all of these things is that they:

o help break down food into forms that are more easily absorbed by the intestines.

o facilitate the absorption of nutrients into the body.

o convert neutral compounds into nutritional powerhouses. One example of this is beta-carotene. Carrots are not, in fact, good for your eyes because of their beta-carotene content, as we are often led to believe. Instead, carrots are good for your eyes because healthy gut flora convert beta-carotene to vitamin A, which is good for your eyes. Vitamin A is extremely important for the human body. Beta-carotene, not quite as much.

o stabilize immune function.

o provide sufficient bulk in the intestines for comfortable and regular bowel movements.

o crowd out unhealthy bacteria that try to sneak into the gut.

o protect the body against toxins that might otherwise enter the bloodstream through inflamed intestinal walls.

o promote healthy serotonin levels in the gut, supporting mental health.

Negative effects of bad gut bacteria

Gut bacteria can also be balanced toward bad guys. This happens when you knock out healthy gut bacteria with antibiotics, as well as when you overfeed bad gut bacteria by consuming inordinate amounts of processed sugar. When bad bacteria chronically overpopulate your gut, the condition is called small intestinal bacterial overgrowth, or SIBO. SIBO is characterized by digestive discomfort, bloating, gas, loss of appetite, and irregular movement of the intestines, which can lead to both constipation and diarrhea. These symptoms make sense when you consider that bad bacteria impair your ability to digest food. They ferment food in ways that good bacteria don't, creating and trapping gases throughout the small intestine.

Bad bacteria also prevent the absorption of nutrients. Instead of converting food into nourishing nutrients like good bacteria do, they overproduce toxic by-products that can sneak into your bloodstream. Since the gut is one of the primary places in which the inside of your body makes contact with the outside, and since it is such a complex barrier, the immune system is highly sensitive to gut health and bacteria populations. I'll return to this point in a moment, but as it turns out, maintaining a healthy gut flora population along with healthy intestinal walls is quite possibly the most important thing you can do to nourish and heal your body, lose weight, and feel good.

Ways to influence gut flora

You have enormous power to influence what populates your gut. One serious risk is taking antibiotics, which kills off good bacteria in the gut. Another is eating processed sugars, which overstimulates bad bacteria. Metabolic distress such as inflammation can also hurt your gut flora population. Even psychological stress impairs gut flora health.

Alternatively, you can improve the state of your gut bacteria by eating *prebiotics* such as onions, garlic, and Jerusalem artichokes, which are the preferred foods of good gut bacteria. You can also eat *probiotics*, which are foods that contain good gut bacteria in and of themselves. Probiotics include a wide variety of fermented foods: sauerkraut, kimchi, kombucha, and full-fat unprocessed yogurt are just a few examples.

Health interaction #2: your intestinal lining

In addition to gut bacteria, food interacts with the intestinal lining itself. Here, in a healthy woman, important nutrients are selectively absorbed into the body and harmful toxins are selectively passed into the colon. If your gut integrity is compromised in any way, however, you may run into serious trouble.

Certain foods actively abrade the intestinal lining. They are irritating, rough, and antagonistic and can make your gut lining permeable over time. *Permeability* in this context means exactly what you think it means: instead of staying outside your body, the contents of your intestines can pass through the damaged lining. In the wake of damage to your intestinal walls, toxic waste from the digestive process, large molecules that otherwise would pass right through your system and everything else your body wants to get rid of can leach into your bloodstream. I don't know about you, but the last thing I want in my bloodstream is the stuff my body would otherwise excrete as feces.

The condition of having a permeable intestinal lining, as unpleasant as it sounds, deserves an equally unpleasant name. Somewhere along the line, the medical community settled on "leaky gut," and we have been stuck with it ever since.

Leaky Gut

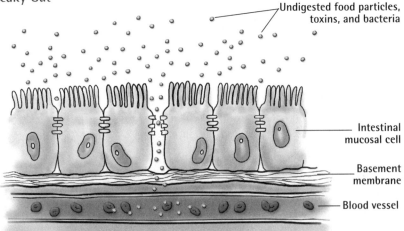

Undigested food particles, toxins, and bacteria

Intestinal mucosal cell

Basement membrane

Blood vessel

Leaky gut means that bad things get into the bloodstream. It also means that the body responds with an immune attack.

Immune activity is ordinarily a good thing. The immune system does not just protect you from disease; it is also responsible for keeping bodily functions running smoothly and cleanly. However, leaky gut can cause so much trouble that it can confuse the immune system with respect to which cells it is supposed to attack. The immune system is specifically designed to target foreign bodies and potential threats and eliminate them. It has sophisticated mechanisms in place for identifying and attacking potential problems. This is how it protects your body from disease. Unfortunately, many toxins that leak into the body as a result of leaky gut resemble human cells. This confuses the immune system into attacking your own healthy cells in addition to the toxins. As the immune system becomes more entrenched in these battles, specific kinds of cells become cemented as targets for attack. This is how individuals develop Hashimoto's thyroiditis, for example. In this case, the body has mistaken thyroid cells for potential threats and as such has learned to target thyroid cells, even though they are an essential part of the healthy human body.

Leaky gut is, therefore, in my and many other health advocates' opinions, the underlying cause of all autoimmune diseases. These include several dozen different diseases, including Hashimoto's thyroiditis, celiac disease, rheumatoid arthritis, multiple sclerosis, lupus, Crohn's disease, Addison's disease, Graves' disease, type 1 diabetes, and ulcerative colitis. In autoimmune conditions, the body attacks human cells because it is confused about who's a good guy and who's a bad guy. How can we blame it?

Autoimmune disease:

A condition in which the body attacks its own cells, often targeting one particular group of cells.

Health interaction #3: the immune response

As a result of toxins getting through the gut barrier and into the body, your immune system can not only get confused, but also send itself into overdrive. This condition is called *systemic inflammation.* Virtually all health professionals now agree that systemic inflammation is the common underlying factor in most noncommunicable diseases, including diabetes, obesity, heart disease, stroke, high blood pressure, high cholesterol, irritable bowel syndrome, asthma, joint pain, eczema, acne, rosacea, osteoporosis, arthritis, depression, anxiety, Alzheimer's, Parkinson's, and many more of the health complications of modern life.

Systemic inflammation occurs when the immune system does not just attack one specific area, but runs rampant throughout the entire body. Inflammation on its own is not always a bad thing. In fact, it's quite good under two specific conditions: when it is short-term, and when it is concentrated in one small area or on one type of tissue. One example in which inflammation is helpful is a physical injury. Say you step on a piece of glass and cut the bottom of your foot. To heal the wound, your body sends repair molecules to the site. Your foot gets red and swollen. It might develop some pus and feel unpleasant for a while. But this happens in just one place and for a short time. Inflammation is the means by which your body heals.

This beneficial process becomes harmful when it no longer has a specific target and occurs throughout the body. When this happens, it's like sending truckloads of security personnel into an already crowded nightclub: they end up causing even worse damage. Your body is doing its best in this case—it is trying. All your security guards are running around fighting all the bad guys they can get their hands on. But there are too many guards, and they cause more panic than they pacify.

Leaky gut causes inflammation, but it is not the only culprit. Stress causes inflammation. High blood sugar and insulin levels cause inflammation. Consuming a lot of omega-6 fat such as vegetable oil causes inflammation. Grains, both whole and refined, have been significantly linked to inflammation. Alcohol, exposure to toxins, poor sleep, and nutrient deficiencies also make it easier for the body to become inflamed. The best way to minimize inflammation is to eat an anti-inflammatory, nutrient-rich healing diet like the *Sexy by Nature* diet and to live a life that is nourishing, stress-reducing, and self-loving.

Silent epidemics: leaky gut and inflammation

While leaky gut is one of the primary contributors to systemic inflammation and plays an important role in the generation of autoimmune disease, both leaky gut and systemic inflammation can go largely unnoticed by the people who have it. You can feel perfectly healthy—or healthy *enough*—and still battle low levels of gut permeability. Signs that indicate inflammation and gut permeability are acne, other skin conditions such as psoriasis, irritable bowel syndrome, constipation, diarrhea, digestive discomfort, joint pain, and abdominal fat, among many others. An important blood marker is C-reactive protein, which indicates (more or less) how much inflammation is present in the body over the course of a month. Large numbers of people do not experience outward symptoms of these problems—*yet*.

Health interaction #4: metabolic hormones

Let's check in. What do we know so far?

○ Healthy gut flora help the body digest food and facilitate the absorption of nutrients.

○ The gut lining needs to be strong and intact to keep toxins out of the body.

○ Inflammation and autoimmune diseases can result from an unhealthy gut.

What happens *after* nutrients have been absorbed into the bloodstream? Your hormones respond by attempting to preserve metabolic fitness. After a meal, two major hormone responses regulate your metabolism. The hormone insulin regulates fat storage, and the hormone leptin regulates appetite. If these processes are disrupted, your ability to eat when you are hungry and stop when you are full and your ability to burn fat will be severely compromised.

Insulin regulates blood sugar

When you eat a meal, insulin is one of the first hormones to react. With all meals (except a meal composed entirely of fat—fat is like a "stealth molecule" with respect to insulin), sugar enters the blood in the form of glucose. Even a couple of teaspoons of sugar in the bloodstream is toxic, so your pancreas gets to work clearing it out *immediately* by secreting insulin. The insulin attaches itself to the sugar molecules and escorts the sugar to fat cells. When it reaches the cells, insulin performs an action similar to knocking on a door and says: "Hello, I have some sugar with me. May I store it, please?"

In a healthy body, the fat cells can hear the knocking and welcome the sugar inside. In a body that has been performing this process on overdrive for long periods, however, the fat cells have a harder time getting up to answer the door. Imagine yourself sitting on the sofa watching TV, having to get up and run to the door every other commercial break. If you did this all day every day, you'd probably get pretty tired of it. This is exactly what happens to your fat cells when they are inflamed, have poor nutrient support, and are constantly at insulin's beck and call: they get tired.

Hormones are messenger molecules. When we hear "hormones," we usually think "sex." This is because the reproductive system is highly involved in cellular messaging. However, other systems in the body utilize these messengers, too. Nearly uncountable hormones are at play in regulating blood sugar, fat metabolism, hunger, sleep, mood, and stress. It goes without saying, then, that the hormonal response a food provokes is one of the most important factors in determining whether it is going to heal you or hurt you.

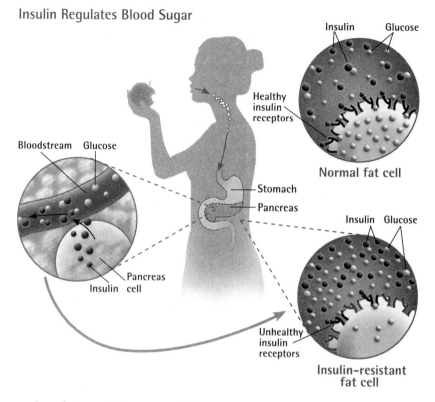

Insulin Regulates Blood Sugar

Insulin Glucose

Healthy insulin receptors

Normal fat cell

Bloodstream Glucose

Stomach

Pancreas

Insulin Glucose

Pancreas
Insulin cell

Unhealthy insulin receptors

Insulin-resistant fat cell

Insulin resistance and its causes

The state of having a difficult time hearing insulin's request is called *insulin resistance*. Insulin resistance is the precursor to diabetes, and it is characterized by a decreased ability of fat cells to detect and store glucose. They become insensitive or resistant to the insulin signal.

Insulin resistance is caused by poor gut and liver health, depleted gut flora, inflammation, overconsumption of sugar-rich processed foods, being overweight, and leptin resistance (see below), all of which put too much pressure on the body's sugar-management and fat-storage mechanisms.

When fat cells can't hear the insulin knocking at their door, the body has to produce more insulin to get through to them. To understand the seriousness of this problem, consider a simple snack such as a banana. When you are healthy, your body might secrete 10 units of insulin to process the glucose in the banana. As you become more and more insulin resistant, however, you'll have to secrete 20 or 30 units to take care of the same banana. The extra insulin produces a louder knock on the fat cells' door.

As cells become insulin resistant, insulin builds up in the bloodstream, which disrupts a wide variety of systems. It inflames the body and depresses healthy immune activity. It also increases testosterone production in the ovaries, which can lead to facial hair growth, acne, low libido, and infertility. Chronically high insulin levels make it supremely difficult, if not impossible, to lose weight.

> Chronically high insulin levels make it supremely difficult, if not impossible, to lose weight.

Leptin determines healthy appetite

Insulin may be the hormone responsible for fat storage, but leptin is the hormone responsible for telling the body how much fat it should store in the first place.

Every fat cell in the human body secretes leptin. This enables the brain to maintain the right "set point." In a healthy body, if you accumulate excess fat, your fat cells pump more leptin into your bloodstream than your brain is programmed for. In response, your brain decreases your appetite, and you crave and eat less. When you have too little leptin in your bloodstream, conversely, your brain makes you crave and eat more. Healthy leptin signaling is the body's natural weight-regulation system. It enables the body to maintain a healthy balance between fat levels and appetite on its own. It maintains a slim waistline on its own. If needed, it dials down your appetite and helps you lose weight on its own. Without healthy leptin signaling, your body compels you to eat more and continually store fat, even if you already have more fat than you need.

Just as your cells can become insulin resistant, they can also become leptin resistant. Like insulin resistance, leptin resistance crops up as a result of chronic overconsumption of unhealthy, inflammatory foods.

Modern diets have done serious damage to leptin signaling. Food today is too stimulating, overriding leptin signals and causing you to eat more than you need. It hijacks your senses, making it impossible for normal hormone signaling to be heard amid the ruckus. Think of a bag of potato chips, for example. You will never get full on a bag of potato chips, even though one bag might contain all the calories you need for a given day. The potato chips become even worse once we consider the fact that they lack the nutrients you need to support a healthy metabolism in the first place. Because of foods like potato chips—or soda, or pizza, or cookies, or even bread—the modern diet offers far too little nutrition and does far too much hormone-overriding damage to allow you to have the smooth and speedy metabolism you would otherwise enjoy.

What about reproductive hormones?

Reproductive health is intimately tied to all the problems I just described. It is hurt by inflammation, bad gut bacteria, leaky gut, and unhealthy insulin and leptin levels. It can be run off-course by even the slightest signs of metabolic distress. Your gut doesn't need ovaries in order to work right, but your ovaries sure as hell need your gut to be in tip-top shape.

Reproductive hormone levels can also be disrupted by the introduction of estrogenic hormones from toxic exposure, such as from BPA (an estrogen-mimicking compound leached from plastic products), or by the consumption of certain estrogenic foods, both of which I discuss below and again in Step 4. These unnatural hormones have the power to interrupt fertility, cause menstrual disorders such as PMS and PMDD, and affect physical and mental health.

The metabolism takeaway

o Overly tasty and addictive foods override your body's natural ability to regulate what you eat. These foods are *designed* to cause you to overeat. This is good news for the food industry, good news for the pharmaceutical industry, and bad news for your body and your wallet.

o Overconsumption of inflammatory, nutrient-poor foods, especially those that are rich in sugar, damages your brain's ability to regulate your appetite.

o Without appetite regulation, overconsumption elevates blood sugar levels, causes sugar to be stored as fat, and leads to insulin resistance, which ultimately causes diabetes, obesity, and more.

A word on macronutrients

Before embarking on a journey through the good foods and the bad, you may find it helpful to learn a bit of the lingo. Health professionals ordinarily separate foods into three broad categories: protein, carbohydrate, and fat. Every food on the planet is composed of one or more of these macronutrients.

Proteins are the building blocks of cells. They make up muscle tissue, and they also comprise neurotransmitters, hormones, and many parts of cells, including DNA. The healthiest protein sources are from animals: beef, bison, chicken, turkey, lamb, pork, game, organ meats, seafood, and eggs. Dairy also contains reasonable amounts of protein. Animal protein is often called *complete* protein. Complete protein contains the whole set of amino acids (the molecules that make up proteins) that the body needs. Nuts and legumes are *incomplete* proteins. They do not have all the amino acids the body needs.

Fat is one of the body's primary fuel sources. Contrary to popular opinion, it is not the demon behind heart disease and obesity. There are many different kinds of fat, some of which cause damage and some of which do not. **Monosaturated fats** include healthy plant fats such as olive oil and avocados. **Polyunsaturated fats** include omega-3 and omega-6 fats and must be held in proper balance in the body in order to maintain good health. Heating polyunsaturated fats to high temperatures and for long periods, as is the case when foods are **deep-fried**, can cause significant inflammation and tissue damage. **Saturated fat** is found primarily in animal products, butter and other dairy, and coconut oil. This type of fat has been vilified, but without good reason. **Trans fat** (also known as hydrogenated or partially hydrogenated fat) is definitely, disastrously unhealthy.

Carbohydrates, like fats, are sometimes healthful and sometimes not. All vegetables, starches, and fruits are healthful carbohydrates. They are natural gifts from the Earth! Grains, legumes, bread, cereal, oats, chips, virtually all snacks, and everything that contains sugar (such as ice cream, cake, soda, and fruit juice) are also carbohydrates, but the unhealthy, processed sort. Corn and grains might seem healthful on first glance—what am I doing lumping them together with ice cream and soda?—but a closer look reveals that they too are unfit for human consumption.

Health trends often prioritize one of these macronutrients over the others. What's better—low-carb or low-fat? No one seems to agree.

I posit a different argument: neither is better. It is not the *type* of macronutrient you eat that makes a difference, but the *quality* of the macronutrient. There are good fats and bad fats. There are good carbohydrates and bad carbohydrates. There are good proteins and less-good proteins. For this reason, I do not focus on macronutrient ratios when I seek optimal health for myself. I do not set rules. Instead, I let my body and my natural cravings dictate what I need at any given time. Certain health conditions may require sharper attention to this issue, such as low carbohydrate for insulin resistance and diabetes, but in general, it is far more important to focus on eating quality proteins, fats, and carbohydrates than it is to focus on eating specific ratios.

The Bad Stuff

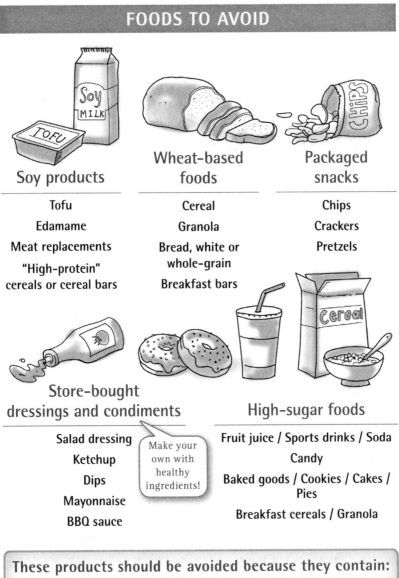

FOODS TO AVOID

Soy products
Tofu
Edamame
Meat replacements
"High-protein" cereals or cereal bars

Wheat-based foods
Cereal
Granola
Bread, white or whole-grain
Breakfast bars

Packaged snacks
Chips
Crackers
Pretzels

Store-bought dressings and condiments
Salad dressing
Ketchup
Dips
Mayonnaise
BBQ sauce

Make your own with healthy ingredients!

High-sugar foods
Fruit juice / Sports drinks / Soda
Candy
Baked goods / Cookies / Cakes / Pies
Breakfast cereals / Granola

These products should be avoided because they contain:

Processing chemicals	Sugar Alcohol	Seed oils Trans fats	Grains Soy and flax

Certain foods fail to meet your body's standard for health. Laboratory inventions, processed sugars, grains, phytoestrogens, and seed oils comprise the bulk of that list. You have no instructions in your DNA for their healthy digestion. When you eat them, your body panics, and they wreak havoc on your otherwise naturally healthy systems. They can damage gut flora, inflame your intestines and the rest of your body, and send hormones out of whack. The result is impaired health and impaired nutrient absorption—phenomena that can send even the healthiest person's body into a panic.

Laboratory inventions

It is already fairly well established that processed foods are bad. They are full of all sorts of chemicals and invented foods that the human body is not designed to handle. Consider a few examples:

○ Folic acid, a B vitamin made solely in laboratories (its natural and digestible form is called folate), has been linked to colon, breast and lung cancer,[9] despite the fact that it continues to be added to bread, cereals, and supplements, promoted as a key component of prenatal nutrition, and listed as a crucial B vitamin.

○ Trans fat (also called hydrogenated or partially hydrogenated fat) in the form of shortening was developed by Procter & Gamble in 1907. The company was looking for an inexpensive alternative to paraffin and beef tallow for making candles and soap. In the end, it made CRISCO, which has been contributing to weight gain, coronary heart disease, insulin resistance, diabetes, and decreased intelligence in newborns for more than 100 years.

○ Certain phosphate additives are used to augment taste, texture, and shelf life in a large proportion of processed foods but are known to cause health problems like rapid aging, weak bones, kidney deterioration, and liver toxicity.

○ Citrus red no. 2 is permitted only for the coloring of orange skins but is toxic to rodents even in modest amounts and causes bladder tumors in rats. Green 3 causes significant increases in bladder and testes tumors in male rats. The FDA recognized Red 3 as a thyroid carcinogen in 1990, though its use is still permitted. Yellow no. 5 is the second most commonly used dye in the U.S. and is linked to hyperactivity in children.[10]

Hundreds if not thousands more examples exist. The problem is twofold: First, these chemicals and invented foods have not been thoroughly studied. All science can tell us for certain is that they are of unnatural origin and that many of them have begun to be correlated with health problems in rodent and human studies. To that end, the best and safest thing you can do for your body is to keep your intake of processed foods and processing chemicals to a minimum.

Second, you may not necessarily know what's in your food. This is a big problem. If you don't know how you are being poisoned, how can you stop it? The solution is to find out what's in it. Read the label. Ask the waiter if you have concerns about the quality of the food at a restaurant. Michael Pollan has a good rule to follow on this score: Do a quick scan of a food label or a chef's ingredient list. If your great-grandmother wouldn't recognize any of the ingredients as food, you shouldn't, either. Sometimes it's impossible to know, or you don't have much of a choice about it. That's okay. Just make sure to consider invented foods as rare treats or expediencies rather than a regular part of your diet.

The laboratory inventions takeaway

Many foods and additives have been invented in laboratories. Not all of these inventions have been investigated for their effects on human health, though most that have are now known to pose serious risks. If your great-grandmother would not recognize an ingredient as food and eat it, then you should not, either.

Sugar

Sugar in all its forms, especially the refined forms such as table sugar and high-fructose corn syrup, is unhealthy for a wide variety of reasons. It is possibly the worst "food" in the Standard American Diet. The human body has not evolved to ingest sugar in the gluttonous portions we do today. Sure, the body was built to process the natural sugars found in whole foods such as fruits and vegetables—and even natural sweeteners like honey and molasses from time to time. Natural carbohydrates are perfectly healthy in reasonable quantities and are some of the best foods for us. But refined sugar in all its glory has *zero* nutrition. *Zero.*

The downsides of sugar

○ **Sugar is actively addictive.** It is directly manufactured to be so. This addictive quality of sugar is the number one cause of overeating, and therefore also of metabolic damage and weight gain.

○ **Sugar hides on nutrition labels.** There are many different chemical forms of sugar, so you might not recognize it on a nutrition label. In fact, most of the foods you consume probably contain several different kinds of sugar. Food companies use this trick to make it seem like there is less sugar in a given food than there actually is. Fructose, glucose, sucrose, maltose, dextrose, saccharose, and any other ingredient that ends in -ose is a sugar. Other common sugars to look out for are maltodextrin, syrup, honey, molasses, agave nectar, evaporated cane juice, cane crystals, treacle, and anything labeled as a sweetener, such as corn sweetener.

o **Sugar spikes insulin levels.** The more sugar you eat, the more your insulin levels rise. The higher your insulin and blood sugar levels rise, the less sensitive you become to both insulin and leptin over time.

o **Sugar promotes the secretion of testosterone from the ovaries.** Insulin is a direct testosterone stimulator. Testosterone disrupts menstrual cycles, causes infertility, and can cause acne, male-pattern hair growth, and male-pattern hair loss.

o **Sugar feeds bad bacteria in the gut.** This leads to SIBO, gut discomfort, bloating, diarrhea, formation of toxins in the gut, and crowding out of good bacteria.

What about fruit juice and other "healthy" beverages?

The food industry might like it if, when you ditched soda, you took up fruit juice and other flavored beverages instead, but you would be wise to avoid all of them. Why? Fruit juice and other "healthy" beverages contain just as much sugar as soda. Conventional orange juice actually has *more* sugar in it than Coca-Cola. Orange juice might edge out Coke in terms of nutritional value because it contains vitamins that facilitate sugar metabolism, but it still contains approximately 30 grams of sugar per cup. Fruit juice is not the healthful alternative we have been duped to believe it is.

Zero- or low-calorie alternatives are not health utopias, either. Diet sodas may have no calories, but they contain hosts of chemicals unfamiliar to the human body. The effects of these chemicals are not yet wholly known, with some studies proclaiming them safe and others calling for cancer-related investigations. Regardless, most health professionals agree that fake sugars confuse the brain. The body responds to the sweetness by priming the brain for a blood sugar surge. When this surge doesn't arrive, the brain feels cheated, and its ability to feel sated from sweet foods diminishes over time. This leads to increased food intake later. In rodent studies, calorie intake and body fat steadily increase on diets that include artificial sweeteners.

A word on alcohol

Alcohol is digested in much the same way sugar is, with even more toxic effects. For one, alcohol is an outright toxin, so when you consume it, your body metabolizes it before everything else. When you have alcohol in your stomach, everything you eat is immediately stored as fat. This is one of the many reasons that alcohol consumption is so strongly linked to weight gain.

Alcohol also disturbs blood sugar levels, increases insulin secretion—especially when combined with the sugars found in mixed drinks—and impairs the action of glucagon, the hormone that promotes fat burning. As a toxin that is processed by the liver, alcohol causes oxidative stress that leads to inflammation, impairs the immune system, promotes overgrowth of bad gut bacteria, and can contribute to irritation of the gut lining. Alcohol is bad for the brain, too: it can kill neurons and hinder signaling in the nervous system.

Heard the news that wine, beer, or some other drink is good for wellness in some specific quantity? Some studies have shown that people who drink on occasion are healthier than those who do not. I strongly suspect that this is because of other lifestyle factors, such as having a healthy social life. Should you raise a glass once in a while? That is your choice! And I hope you will make it peacefully. Life is about living *happily* first and foremost. Alcohol in moderation won't kill you, but it's best to not kid ourselves into thinking that it delivers health benefits.

The sugar takeaway

Sugar provides nothing good while causing a host of problems. More than any other food, sugar has been associated with the rise in obesity, inflammation, and disease over the last several decades. Having trouble losing weight? Making changes in your life? Drop soda. Or fruit juice. Try dropping all flavored beverages. You might be amazed at the enormous power this simple switch has to improve your energy, your skin quality, your weight, and your health.

Grains

Grains—by which I mean all grains, such as wheat, oats, barley, spelt, sorghum, rye, corn, and millet, and all of the products made from them, such as bread, breakfast cereal, and pasta—are a controversial topic these days. Many nutritionists say that whole grains are among the most valuable foods. More discerning nutritionists and scientists, however, have been questioning the pedestal on which we have placed grains for decades. Their number appears to be growing, too.

Much of the current discussion on grains focuses on potential problems with the grain protein gluten. Unfortunately, nutritionists who focus on gluten to the exclusion of other problems with grain products miss the point. It's not just gluten that is cause for concern, and not just for people who test positive for celiac disease. Grains have a lot more harmful potential to go around. They affect all of us and are poor sources of nutrition whether we have celiac disease or not. I know this is not good news since grains are a staple in the Western diet. But in the pursuit of excellent health and radiant sex appeal, you should consider limiting or, better, eliminating grains altogether. It will go a long way toward helping you reach your goals.

Why grains have been put on a pedestal

I have been unable to discern why grains have ever been exalted as health foods. Trust me, I have looked. In an effort to convince you to give them up, I have dug through all the health claims about grains and debunked them. These are the strongest health claims I have found:

Claim #1: Grains contain fiber.

Grains do contain significant amounts of fiber. However, vegetables and fruits contain fiber, too, and eating a moderate amount of fruit and vegetables is more than enough to meet the body's fiber-related needs. Moreover, the kind of fiber in vegetables and fruits is gentler on your gut than the fiber in grains. Vegetables and fruits contain mostly soluble fiber, which feeds good gut bacteria and does not abrade the intestinal lining, while grains contain a significant amount of insoluble fiber, which passes through the body undigested and can abrade the intestinal walls along the way.

Claim #2: Whole grains are a rich source of vitamins and minerals.

Says who? A quick Internet search for "whole grains vitamins and minerals" reveals an entire first page of search results published by whole-grain producers, councils, and advocates—that is, people who make money off the sale of grains. These websites claim that whole grains contain B vitamins, vitamin E, iron, zinc, magnesium, and trace minerals. Granted, grains do contain some B vitamins. They also have a minimal amount of vitamin E and iron—so minimal, in fact, that many health estimates consider the vitamin E in grains to be insignificant. Magnesium is present in grains. Trace minerals such as selenium show up sometimes. But even these small claims dissolve under scrutiny.

First, how much of each of these vitamins is present in grain products depends on the quality of the soil in which the grains are grown, and it's almost certain that whatever flour you consume comes from grain grown on a mineral-depleted stretch of over-farmed soil. Second, many of the vitamins so often espoused as being inherent to grains are not inherent to the grains themselves but are added to flour in a chemical process called *fortification*. This is more problematic than it may seem on the surface. Folic acid, for example, is added to grains, and we have already seen how folic acid has been linked to a variety of cancers. The vitamins added to grain products may not be as helpful as they seem.

Worst of all, grains contain compounds called *phytonutrients,* which actively compete for vitamins in your gut. They bind vitamins to them and carry them away as they are flushed out of your digestive system. Phytonutrients literally steal nutrients you need, making it nearly impossible for your body to absorb any of the minimal nutrition available in grains.

Phytonutrients are part of the bran—the part of the grain that makes it "whole." Can the bran be stripped off grains to make it less toxic? Yes. In fact, we do it on a regular basis to produce refined or white flour, making the bran the only difference between refined and wheat flour. Which is "better" for you? Both are unhealthy in their own ways. Refined flour doesn't have the phytonutrient action inherent in the bran of whole-grain products, but it is devoid of all the nutrients available in grains (unless it's fortified) and spikes blood sugar higher than most other foods, including whole grains.

Claim #3: Grains are an excellent source of protein.

The important questions to ask in response to this claim are: what kind of protein, and how much? Compared to animal products, grains carry much less protein per gram, incomplete protein, and protein that damages the gut.

Most measurements I have found for different types of whole-grain bread grant 4 grams of protein to one slice. A slice of bread usually contains about 100 calories. For 100 calories of tuna, you get 25 grams of protein. That's 600 percent the amount of protein.

The protein in grain products is also incomplete. The term *protein* might sound like it refers to one kind of molecule, but in fact it refers to a whole class of molecules called *amino acids.* When you consume animal protein, every amino acid is present. Your body needs all of them in order to function. Each amino acid has its own special role in maintaining cellular health, building DNA, building neurotransmitters, building muscle, and promoting metabolic fitness and mental health. Grains, however, do not contain all the amino acids. Each type of grain is deficient in its own way.

(Quinoa is a complete protein, but it is not a grain.) Vegetarians and bread lovers need to be careful about their protein sources, or they may miss out on amino acids that are crucial for health.

The types of protein that are present in grains make them devastating for health. Gluten is a grain protein, for one. It has received the most attention and has the most potential to do harm, since it is quite possibly the dominant cause of celiac disease. There are many other harmful proteins in grains that have similar characteristics. Another example is wheat-germ agglutinin, or WGA. Gluten, WGA, and many other grain proteins have the ability to impair digestion, tear holes in the intestinal lining, cause autoimmune diseases, cause allergies, cause weight gain, contribute to insulin resistance, impair gut flora health, and significantly elevate levels of systemic inflammation.

What about rice?

White rice does not contain harmful grain proteins or phytonutrients. This means it does not do any of the damage that grains normally do in the digestive track. It is a fairly innocent food, if high in carbohydrate content and not very nutrient rich. The difference between white rice and brown rice is that white rice has been stripped of the bran, and brown rice still has the bran on it. Brown rice contains more vitamins than white rice and also more fiber, which can be considered good things. The vitamins come at a price, however, because the bran is where the phytonutrients are located.

Claim #4: Grains are a natural part of the human diet.

Grains have *not* always been a part of human history. In fact, grain consumption did not become widespread until approximately 10,000 years ago (or at the earliest 50,000 years ago—not much of a difference in evolutionary terms). This was the time around which people stopped roving the land hunting and gathering food and started settling down to farm and build cities. We have grains to thank for industrialization in large part. But was that necessarily a good thing?

With the advent of agriculture came a host of problems. Anthropologist Jared Diamond of *Guns, Germs, and Steel* fame has argued quite effectively that agriculture directly caused a precipitous decline in human health. If you compare the skeletons of agricultural humans to those of pre-agricultural humans, you find in general (it varies by population) that agricultural humans suffered a decrease in height, an increase in iron-deficiency anemia, an increase in bone lesions caused by disease, and an increase in tooth enamel defects indicative of malnutrition.[11] We cannot say for certain, but it seems as though grains played at least some role in these health problems.

Other factors were at play, but they still pose serious questions about grain consumption. For example, we know part of the problem was that grains pushed other foods such as meat out of the diet. If the problem then was that grains pushed good foods out of the diet, shouldn't we still consider it a problem today? Especially when grain products like bread and pasta take up so much space that we could otherwise devote to nourishing natural foods?

Did humans evolve to eat grains? No. The species has existed in its current form for approximately 2.5 million years. Until approximately 10,000 years ago, humans rarely, if ever, ate grains. Humans were unquestionably best adapted to products that could be hunted or foraged in the wild, including plants and animals. Grains, which require agricultural resources and mills or other means by which to produce flour, were simply inaccessible to humans for the vast majority of human history. So when grain products began emerging as dietary staples in the industrialized world (extant hunter-gatherers do not eat grains), the body reacted poorly. It had never eaten this food before, so it was not built—or at least, wasn't yet built—to peacefully extract nutrition from grains. It didn't have the digestive robustness that a diet full of grains presumably requires.

Have humans rapidly evolved to eat grains in recent history? Probably not. Ten thousand years is 0.4 percent of human history. That would be a lightning-fast adaptation for our DNA. A few people may have benefited from lightning-fast action and developed a great ability to tolerate grains, but they lie far out on the spectrum of tolerance. A few others become radically ill when they eat grains. Most of us fall somewhere in between these two extremes. This in-between space may be the most tragic of all: being here means that we don't know what role grain products may be playing in our health.

As far as health champions go, grains just do not measure up. Their nutrient status is questionable, they contain phytonutrients that block the absorption of vitamins, and the proteins they contain are minimal, incomplete, and highly inflammatory. The real reason grains receive so much emphasis today is that they are so deeply ingrained in Western culture. Grains have been a staple of the human diet since the invention of agriculture, and most of us Westerners can't imagine life without them.

Grain advice

What should you do if you don't know how badly you react to grains? In my opinion, the best thing is to eliminate them from your diet *entirely* for at least three weeks. You can't know what effect they have on you until you stop eating them. One hundred percent elimination is important because even the slightest amount of grain can throw off the whole experiment and cloud the results for someone who has a leaky gut and/or an autoimmune condition. After several weeks of eating grain-free and taking careful notes about the changes you experience, you have the option to try them again. I am willing to bet not only that grains will lose their appeal after weeks without them, but also that the better digestion, clearer skin, clearer head, and greater energy you experience will make you want to leave grains more or less in the dust for good.

The grain takeaway

Bad for your gut, bad for your immune system, and bad for your hormones, grains have a lot of potential to harm you. They impair nutrient absorption, damage intestinal linings, may cause leaky gut, may cause autoimmune conditions, may contribute to systemic inflammation, and may contribute to insulin resistance and diabetes. They almost certainly play a role in being overweight.

The body has no real business with grains. They weren't present for most of human history. Current, traditional cultures that live off the land, like the Kitavans and the !Kung Bushmen, do not consume grain products.

Is it possible that you are one of the lucky ones who aren't bothered all that much by grains? Absolutely. I cannot pretend to know your body. When I eat grains from time to time, nothing bad happens. But even in innocent cases like my own, grains are not optimal. They provide little nutrition, steal nutrition from other foods, act as gut irritants, and provide nutritionally empty calories.

Legumes: the almost-grains

Quite similar to grains is another class of plant foods: legumes. Legumes include all types of beans and peas: sugar snap peas, green beans, chickpeas, soybeans, alfalfa sprouts, kidney beans, black beans, red beans, white beans, lentils, and peanuts all fall into this category.

Legumes are not as bad as grains. They do not contain harmful proteins to the radical extent that wheat products do. They contain more nutrients and are all around more nutritious and less harmful than grains. If you don't have a seriously impaired gut, an autoimmune disease, or a problem with inflammation, you can get away with eating them without incurring significant damage.

On the other hand, legumes contain certain lectins such as phytohemagglutinin that resemble harmful proteins found in grains. As such, they have gut-irritating and inflammatory potential, *especially* for people who already know or suspect that they have autoimmune conditions or leaky gut. These people need to step especially carefully around legumes. Legumes are sometimes associated with leaky gut, inflammation, intestinal discomfort, acid reflux, bloating, gas, diarrhea, growth of bad gut bacteria, and heart disease.

Legumes also contain fairly high amounts of phytonutrients (though not as high as grains), so they have that scary power to leach nutrients out of your intestines. Their phytonutrient content, as well as that of grains, nuts, and seeds, can be neutralized by soaking them in water for several hours before consuming them, yet many of the other potentially toxic components of these foods (such as phytohemagglutinin and gluten) remain.

Phytoestrogens

Most plants contain chemicals called *phytoestrogens*. Breaking this word down reveals exactly what these chemicals are: *phyto* is Greek for "plant" and *estrogen* means, well, "estrogen." The majority of plant foods contain minimal amounts of phytoestrogens. In others, however, phytoestrogens are a problem. Certain legumes, seeds, and nuts contain significant amounts of phytoestrogens. This can be a serious problem when these foods are consumed in large quantities or for women who experience hormonal disruption via any of the conditions I discuss in Step 4.

The most potent offenders are soybeans and flaxseed, which have the potential to disrupt hormone signaling in a large proportion of both women and men. Other legumes, seeds, and nuts, such as chickpeas, beans, and sesame seeds, contain innocent amounts of phytoestrogens for most people, though, again, women who wrestle with any of the hormone health problems discussed in Step 4 may want to step carefully around them.

What phytoestrogens do

Phytoestrogens are tricky. They take up space on the body's estrogen receptors (the sites responsible for estrogen activity), but they are not as powerful as natural estrogen. What this means is that they *act* like estrogen and take up as much space as estrogen, but they do not effectively perform estrogen's functions.

In most women, consuming soy and flax leads to an accumulation of too much estrogen in the body. Phytoestrogens pile up on top of one another and create a hyper-estrogenic environment, inducing PMS, menstrual cramps, and mood swings. In other women, particularly those with hormone deficiency problems, soy and flax consumption can lead to too *little* estrogen in the body. In this case, phytoestrogens displace estrogen at receptor sites, fail to perform proper estrogenic function, and cause the opposite kind of hormonal imbalance. Instead of being overly "feminized" by estrogen and picking up menstrual disorders, these women are "masculinized" and pick up symptoms of low estrogen, such as acne and male-pattern hair growth and hair loss.

In many women, phytoestrogens don't make much of a difference. Unfortunately, there's no hard and fast way to tell how much phytoestrogens will affect you until you remove them from your diet. Because you can tip one way or the other, chances are good that eliminating soy and flax and limiting nuts will result in a better hormone balance. Having too much estrogen is a common problem, and phytoestrogens can play a significant role in symptoms such as PMS and mood swings. Overcoming both estrogen

Dietary sources of soy

You might think that there is no soy in your diet because you do not eat tofu or edamame. If you eat anything that comes in a bag or box or has gone through a factory, however, chances are quite good that there is a *significant* amount of soy in your diet.

Most processed foods contain soy protein isolate, soybean oil, soy lecithin, or a combination of these products. Soy is a multitalented plant, and its protein has binding properties that make it ideal for use in many foods. Soybean oil is also fairly flavorless, so many processed foods rely on it as a fat source. Many breakfast cereals (especially the ones that claim to be a good source of protein), cookies, chips, energy bars, snack foods, candies (especially the chewy varieties), chewing gum, chocolate bars, salad dressings, mayonnaise, pasta sauces, other sauces and condiments, frozen dinners, instant meals, and nearly all processed Asian foods have soy in them.

dominance (under the heading "PMS") and estrogen deficiency (under "Infertility") is covered extensively in Step 4.

The phytoestrogen takeaway

Hormone balance is one of the most crucial elements of a woman's health. Period. Regardless of how your body personally reacts to the consumption of phytoestrogens, it is always the case that the more potent phytoestrogens you eat, the more your body's natural estrogenic rhythm is being disrupted. Soy and flax are the worst offenders. Nuts, seeds, beans, chickpeas, and other legumes follow.

BPA

BPA, a chemical found in plastic products (especially heated plastics) and in the linings of aluminum cans, acts as an estrogen in the bloodstream. Its chemical structure is different from that of plant estrogens such as soy and flax, and its true effects on the body are unknown. However, rats that are fed BPA experience decreased fertility. Their offspring are at greater risk for reproductive disorders and have even been reported to have cystic ovaries. For both your own health and the health of your children, avoiding BPA should be a fairly high priority.

Some plastic products are now being made BPA-free. This is a good thing. It helps. But other estrogenic compounds remain. Aluminum cans are also lined with BPA unless specifically stated otherwise. For this reason, it is safest to stick to glass or metal water bottles and cookware. It is also safest to refrain from microwaving plastic cookware or from drinking hot beverage out of plastic mugs. It won't kill you to use plastics or to eat food from cans from time to time, and a healthy liver can usually healthfully process BPA, but it may be better to err on the side of caution.

BPA is also found on receipts. If you work with receipts as a cashier or an accountant, consider wearing protective gloves.

Seed Oils

Seed oils are the toxic foods that cause the most furrowed brows when I mention them. What's a seed oil, and what's it got to do with anything?

Any kind of oil or fat made from a seed is a seed oil. The list is long: vegetable oil, canola oil, peanut oil, soybean oil, rapeseed oil, corn oil, cottonseed oil, linseed oil, flax oil, grapeseed oil, hemp oil, safflower oil, sesame oil, sunflower oil, and wheat germ oil.

The problem with seed oils is that they are completely unnatural. Sure, they come *from* nature. But just like grains, they require significant processing in order to be ingestible, and that processing makes them radically unhealthy.

Seed oils are alarmingly recent additions to the human diet; like grains and sugar, no culture outside of industrialized ones consumes them. Seed oils were virtually unheard of in the American diet until scientists and the U.S. government began promoting them as cholesterol-lowering foods in the 1970s. These oils may lower cholesterol in small amounts, but that says nothing of the real damage they cause to the cardiovascular system and other systems in the body. They are major culprits in cardiovascular disease, and lowering cholesterol on the back end does little to counteract the damage that these oils do up front.

Seed oils are the most common fats in the American diet. This makes them the sneakiest and most sinister of all the food toxins. Don't get me wrong—all the foods on this list have pretty powerful consequences—but seed oils are downright shady in addition to being bad. They are found in nearly every product that comes in a package and are likely used to cook every dish on a typical restaurant's menu. Why? Seed oils are cheap, are tasteless (which makes them compatible with a wide variety of foods), and have been manufactured to have longer shelf lives, a process that explicitly removes any antioxidants inherent to the seeds. Does that sound like something you want to put in your body?

How to tell which plant fats are safe and which are harmful

The trick to knowing right away whether a plant fat is good for you is to consider whether you could find and easily consume this kind of fat in the wild. For example, olives and avocados are quite safe to consume. Coconut is another example. These fats require little processing in order to be consumed in pretty high quantities. You can pluck them right off a tree and eat to your heart's desire.

To consume canola oil, however, you'd have to press hundreds of seeds to yield the tiniest amount of oil. This high level of processing is impossible in the wild. Ancient cultures would never have gone (and current foraging cultures would never go) to the trouble of grinding so many seeds to obtain a teaspoon or two of oil. Making anything resembling modern seed oils would have been quite difficult in ancient history. And even if ancestral humans had made seed oils, they would not have experienced the toxifying effects of industrial processing. The human body is not wired to consume high quantities of these oils, of that there is no question.

What's so dangerous about seed oils: omega-6 fat

Seed oils are dangerous because they have been stripped of their antioxidant potential, for one. More importantly, however, they contain omega-6 fat, which is toxic in high doses.

Omega-6 fat is healthy to a certain point, but its prevalence in the American diet has caused serious problems. Most health professionals call for no more than 4 percent of the diet to be composed of omega-6 fat, yet the average American obtains 9 percent of calories from omega-6 fat. Even more startling is that in the 1960s, omega-6 fat comprised about 8 percent of fat tissue in the average American body. The most recent estimates put it at around 23 percent of fat tissue today.[12] Intake of omega-6 fat has more than doubled, and its levels in the human body have tripled.

Omega-6 fat is tied to elevated rates of liver disease, atherosclerosis (a type of heart disease), obesity, allergies and asthma, irritable bowel syndrome, ulcerative colitis, mental illness, depression, anxiety, cancer, and Alzheimer's disease. A wide swath of studies across different countries and research groups has shown that high–seed oil diets raise death rates by 50 to 350 percent.[13] Even at the low end, 50 percent is an enormous increase in mortality.

Why so bad? First, seed oils as omega-6 fat rancidize easily—so easily, in fact, that most of the seed oils you consume are likely rancid. Rancidification occurs when seed oil is exposed to higher temperatures and brighter light sources than might readily occur in nature. The heat and light of modern kitchens render the molecules unfamiliar to the human body, making them actively harmful. Significant damage can occur even if the oil is sitting on the countertop in a clear bottle. Imagine how rancid these oils become when heated on the stovetop or deep-fried at extreme temperatures over minutes, hours, and days in restaurants after having been stored in clear plastic bottles for months or years? Deep-fried food is almost always made with rancid seed oils.

Rancidity is the chemical decomposition of fats that creates reactive oxygen species and inflammation upon entering the body.

Reactive oxygen species damage organ tissue, wrinkle skin, and damage DNA. Too much reactive oxygen in the body has been linked to systemic inflammation, cardiovascular disease, cancer, and Alzheimer's disease.

Second, and perhaps most importantly, omega-6 fat is explicitly inflammatory. Is this a bad thing? Not necessarily. The body uses omega-6 fat as an inflammatory molecule. As discussed earlier in Step 2, inflammation is important. We need omega-6 fat in order to survive and to perform immune system functions. It is important to consume some level of omega-6. Too much omega-6, however, creates systemic inflammation. This largely accounts for why omega-6 fat is linked to so many health problems: it is one of the causes of the inflammation crisis.

Fortunately, the inflammatory properties of omega-6 fat have a counterweight: the anti-inflammatory properties of omega-3 fat. Omega-3 fat helps calm the immune system after stressful events (you can find more on this in the section on seafood). An imbalance between these two fats—which Americans definitely have, clocking in at a ratio of about 15:1 instead of 2:1[14]—is perhaps the most insidious contributor to systemic inflammation.

Omega-6 fat is found primarily in seed oils, nuts, and industrially raised animal products. Omega-3 fat is found in fish, seafood, and grass-fed, naturally raised animal products. Because dietary sources of omega-3 are rare, and consuming high levels of these kinds of fats is not ideal anyway, the best way to achieve balance is to keep omega-6 and seed oil consumption to a minimum.

Omega-6 fat and nuts

Omega-6 fat is the primary constituent of almost all nuts except macadamias, which provides fair impetus to keep nuts in the diet to a minimum as an occasional snack. Why eat nuts (in reasonable quantities) and not seed oils? Aside from being so easy to overdo, seed oils are worse because they have almost definitely been rancidized, which increases their inflammatory potential.

The seed oil takeaway

Seed oils such as canola, vegetable, and soybean oil are unnatural products that the body does not recognize. They cause significant damage, contributing to oxidative stress and systemic inflammation in the body. Limiting seed oils soothes inflammation and may be one of the greatest boons to healthy immune function, weight loss, hormone health, and overall healing.

Seed oils are harmful largely because they are composed of omega-6 fat. Omega-6 fat is good for the body in small quantities, but in excess overstimulates inflammatory processes. Fortunately, eliminating them is not the only way to reduce inflammation. Omega-6 fat is balanced by omega-3 fat in the body. Adding some omega-3 to your diet can be quite helpful for health and weight loss. Omega-3 fat is found primarily in fish, seafood, and grass-fed, naturally raised animal products.

Nature's
Sexifying Powerhouses

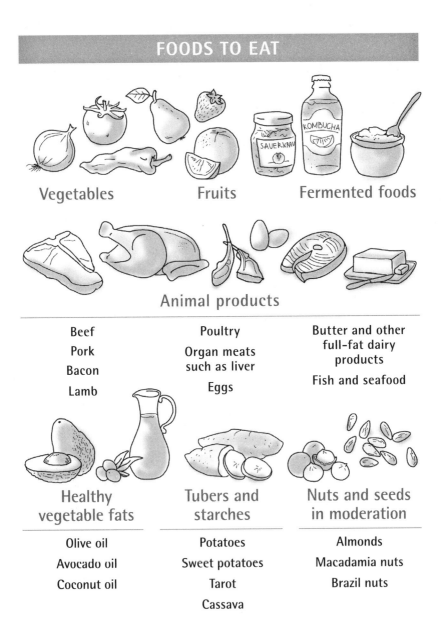

FOODS TO EAT

Vegetables   Fruits   Fermented foods

Animal products

Beef	Poultry	Butter and other full-fat dairy products
Pork	Organ meats such as liver	
Bacon		Fish and seafood
Lamb	Eggs	

Healthy vegetable fats   Tubers and starches   Nuts and seeds in moderation

Olive oil	Potatoes	Almonds
Avocado oil	Sweet potatoes	Macadamia nuts
Coconut oil	Tarot	Brazil nuts
	Cassava	

The list of foods better left on grocery store shelves probably seems pretty long. Daunting, even. Not only does it include the usual suspects, such soda and French fries, but it also includes some things you've been told your whole life are healthy! Even whole grains are on the list. Is there anything left to eat? Can your diet be satisfying at all?

To be honest, I can't think of a more satisfying diet than the *Sexy by Nature* diet. Grains may be hard to give up at first, but the foods recommended in the *Sexy by Nature* diet are way more exciting than the foods it excludes. The excluded foods lead to weight gain, acne, fatigue, poor sleep, poor mental health, and disease. The included foods, on the other hand, do just the opposite: they heal, energize, slim the waistline, and support mental health. They are also hearty and satisfying! *Sexy by Nature* not only gives you the freedom but also *actively encourages* you to eat as much as you crave, to eat unlimited servings of meat, and to go wild with butter, lard, bacon, eggs, cream, and other decadent natural fats. Guacamole, coconut parfaits, mashed potatoes, mango smoothies, and blueberry tarts are a few other treasures of nature's sexifying powerhouses. In this book, just about any food sourced from the wild is fair game.

Vegetables

Vegetables are rich in antioxidants and vitamins. I don't need to tell you this, but the endorsement bears repeating: vegetables are awesome. In fact, vegetable-rich diets have repeatedly been linked to lower incidences of disease and better immune system function, as well as reduced risks for heart disease and cancer. Vegetables are anti-inflammatory, largely because they are rich sources of antioxidants such as vitamin C, vitamin E, and beta-carotene. *All* vegetables are not just fair game, but kick-ass in my book. And *delicious* as well. There is almost no such thing as too many vegetables.

The vegetables most worthy of your attention are green. They include spinach, kale, chard, lettuce, collard greens, broccoli, and Brussels sprouts. Dark green, leafy vegetables as a class are the most nutrient dense of all plant foods. In terms of nutrient density, they knock fruits out of the ballpark. For example, one serving of broccoli has 150 percent the vitamin C of an orange.

Vegetables contain minute amounts of protein and fat but are mostly carbohydrate in the form of glucose. Does this mean that they spike blood sugar levels unhealthfully? Hardly! Vegetables are inherently low in calories. They also contain large quantities of fiber, which slows the insulin response.

Eating vegetables won't fill you up unless you pair them with denser calorie sources such as olive oil, avocados, or a steak. Your body needs healthy energy density—that is, calories—in order to experience fullness. This point is quite important. For a meal to be satisfying and to deliver the nutrients your body needs, it should not rely wholly on vegetables but should include lots of healthy fats and protein sources, too. Moreover, many of the vitamins found in vegetables are fat soluble. They can only be absorbed into your bloodstream when there's fat in your meal. This is partly why fat is such an important part of this diet. Eat your vegetables with fat, and every cell in your body will thank you.

Some green caveats

Just because greens are uniquely nutrient dense does not mean that your diet should consist solely of greens. Healthy balance is the name of the game, since all foods can become toxic when eaten to extremes. Greens, for example, while being packed full of vitamins C, E, and K, also contain a class of compounds called goitrogens, which, when overconsumed (especially when raw or fermented), can inhibit thyroid function. Greens are also high in fiber, which can be problematic for people who have very sensitive guts. The best way to eat your veggies is to emphasize green but also to rotate the color palette of your plate. Greens, oranges, reds, purples, yellows...a rainbow of vegetables cannot steer you wrong.

Some exceptions to the super-low-calorie rule for vegetables are the sweeter vegetables such as beets and acorn squash. You can guess which vegetables are denser sources of carbohydrate almost solely by how sweet they taste. If they taste like fruit, then they probably have as much sugar in them as fruit. These sweeter, more carbohydrate-rich vegetables should not be avoided just because they have more calories or carbohydrates in them, however. Their carbohydrate content is still quite low and definitely within the healthy range. I mention this only because health issues such as diabetes can be mitigated by limiting carbohydrates in the diet.

Starches: potatoes, sweet potatoes, and more

Starches such as potatoes, sweet potatoes, yams, yucca root, tarot, and cassava are generally classed as vegetables, but they deserve their own mention. Why? Because they contain significant amounts of carbohydrate, starch, and soluble fiber.

Starches are carbohydrate rich, but that is not a bad thing in and of itself. Spiking insulin levels, in fact, is not inherently bad. Insulin metabolism is healthy as long as it occurs in the context of meals, natural foods, and a healthfully functioning metabolic system. Usually only in the case of metabolic damage and inflammation do carbohydrates contribute to insulin resistance. Having at least a little bit of carbohydrate in your diet is necessary for healthy thyroid and reproductive systems, and starches are one way women can happily and healthfully meet that need.

Two components of potatoes, sweet potatoes, and other starches make them great sources of carbohydrate. First, starches contain soluble fiber. Soluble fiber is a great food for gut bacteria, which helps improve insulin and other metabolic signaling. Second, the nature of starch safeguards against insulin problems: starch is a type of molecule that slows carbohydrate metabolism and keeps blood sugar and insulin levels steady.

Fruit

Fruit is rich in fiber, antioxidants, and vitamins and is a dense source of carbohydrate. It is another excellent way to meet carbohydrate needs, as well as to satisfy your sweet tooth. You may not want to make your whole diet one of bananas and apples, but fruit is a perfectly natural and healthy way to obtain nutrients, energy, and calories.

Much like starches, fruit has natural properties that make it somewhat impervious to blood sugar problems the way processed foods never can be. First, fruit is made up of more fructose—as opposed to glucose—than other carbohydrates found in the wild, such as starchy vegetables. Glucose and fructose are digested differently. Whereas glucose goes into the bloodstream and immediately becomes blood sugar, fructose must first be processed by the liver, which prevents blood sugar levels from spiking precipitously. Second, fruit contains not just fiber but a host of vitamins and antioxidants, the most important being vitamin C. These vitamins help insulin metabolism run smoothly and prevent blood sugar from becoming a problem when fruit is consumed in moderation.

To buy organic or not?

As I write this book, I earn a salary below the Boston poverty line. Do I eat organic produce? I don't, actually. I can't afford it, and that's okay. If my rent weren't so high, I would visit local farms, pick my own produce, and delight in a bounty of local and organic fruits and vegetables. That is not a luxury I shell out for, however. I have accepted it as a part of my life. The point is to do your best. Organic fruits and vegetables do not have pesticides, industrial solvents, food additives, or polishers such as wax applied to them. They have more vitamins than non-organic fruits and vegetables. They are definitely better for you and usually better for the Earth than their non-organic counterparts. But if you can't eat them, it's all right. You can still benefit from the produce available in your price range, especially if you peel it.

A brief note on skins

Most modern nutritionists are obsessed with the skins of vegetables and fruits. "All the nutrients are in the skin!" they proclaim. "Make sure to eat the skin!" "You have to buy organic so you can eat the skin!" I happen to have the complete opposite opinion. Here's why:

The skin is the part of the plant that defends it against being eaten. Like most things in the animal kingdom (with a few exceptions, such as fruits that want their seeds to be carried far away), plants do not want to be eaten. They want to survive. Skin therefore acts as a barrier against predators. Vegetable skins and fruit peels do the same exact thing that the bran of grain products does: they contain harmful phytonutrients, those chemicals that prevent nutrient absorption. For this reason, even though a fair amount of the nutrition in plant foods is found in the skin, that nutrition gets flushed out of your system right along with the skin anyway. The skin has the added detriment of being contaminated by pesticides, germs, and all the other nasty stuff it encounters on its way to your refrigerator. For these reasons, peeling fruits and vegetables keeps toxins to a minimum, prevents anti-nutrients from stealing your vitamins, and maintains the significant vitamin and mineral power of the fruits and vegetables. If you really love your peels, make sure to buy organic or at least to wash them thoroughly.

Beef and meat from other four-legged critters

Contrary to popular opinion, beef products are some of the most healthful foods available. Saturated fat is not inherently unhealthy, and red meat is not going to give anyone cancer. Perhaps I should restate those facts: saturated fat is not inherently unhealthy, and red meat is not going to give anyone cancer. Both have been wrongfully conflated and mixed up with studies on heart disease.

The skinny on saturated fat and heart disease

Saturated fat has been linked to heart disease, inflammation, cancer, and just about every other disease you can think of. If it's bad, someone somewhere out there has said that saturated fat is to blame.

However, in 2010, a review in the *American Journal of Clinical Nutrition* demonstrated that there wasn't enough proof to link saturated fat to either heart disease or stroke. This meta-analysis involved 21 studies and nearly 350,000 people. These are big, statistically powerful numbers.

While saturated fat elevates LDL cholesterol, it does not elevate triglycerides (highly inflammatory molecules) the same way that carbohydrates do. Most people increase their carbohydrate intake when they reduce their saturated fat intake. It is a trade-off. Unfortunately for these people, it is not a beneficial trade-off, since the increased carbohydrate intake (presumably of poor quality) leads to elevated triglyceride levels, whereas leaving saturated fat in the diet does not have negative health effects. Saturated fat may not be the best fat, but as just one component of many in a natural diet, it does no significant harm, especially if it keeps consumption of less-healthy alternatives to a minimum.

Beef, lamb, bison, pork, game, and all other ruminant products (ruminant is the name for an animal that grazes) are all healthful sources of complete protein that are replete with vitamins and minerals. Truly. They are not devoid of nutrition. On the contrary, animal products contain ample vitamins and minerals that are necessary for bodily function.

Beef is one of the richest sources of B vitamins, for example. Do plant products contain B vitamins? Yes. But they do not contain as much as animal products do, *and,* most importantly, you can't obtain vitamin B_{12}, which is crucial for survival, from plants. Beef is also rich in iron, zinc, potassium, copper, selenium, manganese, phosphorus, and vitamin E.

Poultry

Poultry is a good source of protein. Chicken is a rich source of vitamin B$_3$, or niacin, as well as the trace mineral selenium. Turkey is also a dense source of B vitamins. However, both chicken and turkey contain smaller amounts of most of the minerals found in animal products—such as iron and zinc—than beef. Poultry also has higher concentrations of omega-6 fat than beef does, which makes it a less-optimal source of protein than beef, pork, bison, lamb, and other ruminants.

Don't fall into the trap of thinking that poultry is healthier just because it's leaner. The most important factor is the *quality* of the fat. The only case in which the leanness of a given animal product might make it healthier is with industrially raised animals. Toxins are primarily stored in the fat of the animals, so choosing white meat or leaner cuts of meat can help you avoid the disadvantages of industrially raised meat.

Organ meat

"Ugh, really?" is the response I normally get to this one. "Organ meat? Like heart and kidneys and stuff?"

"Yeah!" I reply enthusiastically, pretending for the thousandth time that I am surprised by the skepticism I have encountered.

Most people can stomach the fact that I eat meat for breakfast. Liver, though, is always a little harder for them to wrap their heads around.

I eat liver regularly not only because I find it delicious, but also because it is possibly the most nutrient-dense food. Liver is packed with enough vitamin A to nourish a family of five for a month. In fact, it provides so much vitamin A that you have to be careful not to eat too much. Carrots and other plants have zero units of vitamin A, instead carrying only its weaker precursor, beta-carotene. Lean muscle meat has 40 units of vitamin A. Calf liver? 53,400 units.[15]

Animal fats and industrialization

I mentioned earlier that you should do your best to eat organic plant products whenever you can. The same principle more or less applies to animal products. The difference between plants and animals, however, is that it is even more important to seek out the good stuff when it comes to animal products. The differences between industrial and truly natural animal products can be striking.

For virtually all of Earth's history, animals have eaten and existed off of their natural food sources. Cows ate grass, not soy, corn, grain, or Snickers bars (this is not a joke; it happened in 2012 during a corn shortage). Chickens ate insects and grasses. Fish ate plankton, algae, and krill.

Deviations from these natural diets have caused real problems in the modern world. Cows, pigs, chickens, fish, and other farmed animals are raised on the cheapest foods manufacturers can get their hands on: grain, soy, corn, and edible leftovers from farming processes. Animals raised on these products are often sick because these foods aren't a part of their natural diets. This means that they need to be pumped full of antibiotics in order to stay disease free. Their being sick, aside from being unpleasant and sad in and of itself, does not spell good things for the level of nutrition available in their meat. There are three important effects of poor diet on industrially raised animals: 1) the vitamin and mineral content is decreased, 2) the toxin load is increased, and 3) fat profiles are skewed toward inflammatory omega-6 and away from anti-inflammatory omega-3. Better for the animals and better for you, eating meat from local farms, if you can, is an excellent way to promote wellness.

Vitamin K is an often underappreciated vitamin that promotes the growth of strong bones, helps blood clot effectively, prevents calcification of arteries, and provides possible protection against liver disease. It comes in two forms, both of which are crucial for health. **Vitamin K_1** is available in kale, spinach, broccoli, and all other leafy greens. Vitamin K_1 can be converted to vitamin K_2, but at a low rate. **Vitamin K_2** is available in natto, fermented or aged cheeses, egg yolks, grass-fed butter, and grass-fed chicken and meat livers.

Liver is also the best source of all the B vitamins and is a great source of copper, iron, and vitamins A, D, E, and K. Liver is especially powerful when it is from grass-fed cows because grass-fed liver contains vitamin K_2, which is essential for a healthy metabolism, healthy heart, strong bones, and clear skin.

Liver is the most nutrient-dense organ meat, though heart and kidneys are also powerful options. Any part of the animal, really, is fair game. And nearly any part of the animal that is not simple muscle tissue (the stuff we ordinarily eat) is going to have more or at least unique nutrition in it. This makes basic biological sense: more nutrition resides in organ and essential tissues because they perform complex functions that are essential to life. Muscle tissue, not quite as much.

There is one final bonus to organ meats: because Americans have learned to reject them even while the rest of the world prizes them highly, they are some of the cheapest foods on the market. This makes them arguably the best sources of sexy nutrition for a natural but scrappy woman.

Fish and seafood

Fish and seafood are some of the healthiest sources of dietary protein and fat. Salmon is a particularly vitamin-rich food and contains high levels of vitamin D as well as vitamin A, all the B vitamins, potassium, phosphorus, calcium, magnesium, and selenium.

One of the primary reasons seafood is so good for the body is that seafood is the richest source of omega-3 fat. You'll recall from the section on seed oils that omega-3 fat is important because it acts as a counterbalance against omega-6 fat. Omega-3 fat is explicitly anti-inflammatory and has been demonstrated to have enormous health benefits across a wide variety of health conditions for this reason. Omega-3 fat has been associated with better mental health, improved cardiovascular health, lower triglyceride levels, increased fertility, and increased intelligence of newborns. It can help in overcoming inflammatory conditions such as rheumatoid arthritis and asthma and in reducing symptoms of mental health disorders such as depression, anxiety, ADHD, and Alzheimer's.

Worried about mercury? Don't sweat it. Here's why: mercury is toxic, but its toxic effects are mitigated by the mineral selenium, which is present in nearly all seafood. If you are still concerned—and really, with the level of toxins found in today's oceans, that fear is reasonable—focus on eating smaller fish. The smaller a fish is, the less mercury it will have in its tissues, since mercury builds up in higher levels of the food chain. Focus on sardines, herring, and salmon, and forgo larger fish such as tuna and swordfish.

Natural animal lingo

For beef products, the words you want are "pasture-raised," "grass-fed," or "grass-finished." Chicken and turkey should be "pasture-raised" as well. Fish should be "wild-caught." Be careful not to be duped by a meat product labeled "natural." "Natural" only means that no additives or preservatives were introduced to the meat after it was processed. It has virtually nothing to do with the quality of the animal product itself.

If you eat industrially raised meat products, it's okay. They won't kill you. In order to minimize omega-6 fat and toxin load while eating industrial meat, your best bet is to go with leaner cuts, since most of the toxins in animal products are found in the fat. This is not a concern with pasture-raised and truly natural animal products. In that case, the fat is supremely healthful and should be liberally consumed.

The skinny on cholesterol and heart disease

Much like saturated fat, cholesterol has been wrongfully accused. Cholesterol is a healthy part of normal bodily processes. Depending on how healthy you are, your body produces far more cholesterol than you eat—up to ten times as much. The body produces cholesterol for many reasons, yet one of the primary reasons is as a response to inflammation and tissue damage. This is a crucial point: the body produces cholesterol to help damaged areas. If we didn't inflame our bodies and our arteries in the first place, then our bodies wouldn't create so much cholesterol in response. Eating cholesterol-rich foods is not to blame for heart disease. Inflammation is.

Cholesterol is a good guy caught in the inflammatory crossfire. Its presence in LDL form indicates that something may be wrong, but *eating* cholesterol does not cause the problem. In fact, a 2011 study out of Norway, published in the *Journal of Evaluation in Clinical Practice*, followed 52,000 men and women over ten years and found higher cholesterol levels in the blood to be associated with a lower risk of death in women of all ages.[16]

Eggs

Eggs are supremely healthful foods and great sources of protein and fat. Contrary to popular opinion (again!), a diet rich in eggs will not cause heart disease. Consuming cholesterol has not been sufficiently linked to heart disease in medical literature; in fact, many studies published in the last few years have demonstrated that cholesterol is actively beneficial for increasing a woman's lifespan. I suggest that you take a moment to meditate on that fact, and then wake up tomorrow morning and eat an omelet.

Eggs contain the building blocks for an entire organism, so they contain a wide array and a high concentration of nutrients. Some of my more brilliant health-advocate friends consider eggs nutritional powerhouses that should be eaten daily. Eggs are rich in choline, which is crucial for liver health and quite rare. They also have plenty of calcium, iron, phosphorus, zinc, copper, manganese, selenium, potassium, many of the B vitamins (including B_5, B_6, B_{12}, and folate), and vitamins A, D, E, and K. Most importantly, the vast majority of nutrition from eggs is contained in the yolk. Contemporary nutritionists demonize egg yolks because they contain saturated fat and cholesterol, yet both saturated fat and cholesterol are quite healthy. Egg yolks can and should play a significant role in your regular eating habits.

Healthy vegetable fats: olive, avocado, and coconut

Why these plant fats and not others? As explored earlier, olives, avocados, and coconuts are easily found in large quantities in the wild. You could pull plenty of olives off a branch, for example, or eat whole avocados at a time. This is not the case with seed oils, which are high in omega-6 fat. Olive oil is mostly monosaturated fat, which has been linked to decreased risks of breast cancer, heart disease, and stroke. Avocados are also composed primarily of monosaturated fat. Both contain antioxidants, specifically vitamin E, which helps prevent oxidative damage and can protect against diabetes. Monosaturated fat is arguably the healthiest kind of fat.

Coconut oil and other coconut products are composed of saturated fat, but that does not make them inherently unhealthful. In fact, coconut oil is a special kind of saturated fat called a *medium-chain fatty acid,* and it has unique fuel-burning and anti-inflammatory capacities. Many health advocates and scientific theorists believe that coconut oil aids in weight loss because of its fat-burning properties and vitamin content.

Coconut oil is great for mitochondria, the parts of your cells responsible for making and burning energy. It helps fight infections because of the antimicrobial properties of lauric acid, a fatty acid that is present in coconut oil in high amounts. And it's great for supporting detoxification, which can help a wide variety of conditions, such as Alzheimer's disease. Coconut products are rich in potassium, selenium, calcium, magnesium, and vitamins B_1, B_2, B_3, and B_9 (folate).

Fermented foods

One of the most powerful things you can do for your health is to improve the health of your gut flora. This boosts immune function, mental health, insulin sensitivity, hormone balance, and just about every primary category of health you can think of. It is impossible to understate the importance of healthy gut bacteria.

The first important step in improving the health of your gut is to eliminate gut irritants such as grains, legumes, and dairy. The second is to add foods that promote gut health by enriching your gut flora population. One way to do so is to take probiotic supplements, which introduce certain strains of healthy bacteria to your gut. The problem with supplements, however, is that gut bacteria are infinitely diverse, and a truly healthy gut may require different bacteria than the ones available in the particular supplement you choose to take. Fortunately, you can cultivate a wide variety of bacterial strains in your gut by consuming a wide variety of bacteria-containing foods. These are all of the fermented foods, and they include sauerkraut, kimchi, natural, unpasteurized, full-fat yogurt, kefir, natto, kombucha (fermented tea), and other fruits and vegetables that have undergone fermentation processes.

Select nuts in moderation

Nuts and seeds are natural foods that are tolerated well by many people. More often than not, however, they are composed primarily of omega-6 fat, so it's best to limit them in your diet.

They also contain large amounts of phytonutrients, those nutrient blockers that are found in high quantities in grains. And most of them are fairly high in phytoestrogens as well. A handful of nuts or seeds here and there is no problem. A tub of almond butter every day would be another story.

Nonetheless, nuts are fairly nutrient dense, and some of them are uniquely healthful. My favorites are almonds, walnuts, macadamia nuts, and Brazil nuts. Almonds are rich in vitamin E, magnesium, phosphorus, calcium, and zinc, and while they contain a significant amount of omega-6, it is balanced by a fair amount of monosaturated fat. Walnuts are composed of more omega-6 fats but have a better omega-6 to omega-3 ratio than other nuts, and they are rich in calcium, iron, zinc, and vitamin B_6. Macadamia nuts are arguably the most healthful of all nuts and have the highest proportion of monosaturated fat. They are rich in thiamine and contain calcium, phosphorus, potassium, sodium, selenium, iron, and B vitamins. Though Brazil nuts are composed primarily of omega-6 fat, they are the richest natural source of selenium; eating just two a day is equivalent to taking a selenium supplement.

If you are going to eat nuts, it is important to buy them fresh, not baked in any kind of oil or roasted. As with the liquid omega-6 fat in seed oils, heat can turn nuts rancid, and eating rancid foods destroys tissue and causes oxidative damage in the body.

Because nuts are tasty, dense nuggets of fat, they are fairly high in calories. For this reason, people who snack on nuts might find that they have a hard time losing weight or feeling appropriately hungry at mealtimes. It's easy to overeat nuts, especially when they are salty and roasted and perfect for crunching on a stressful day. Keep the nuts to a minimum, and be wary of how easy it is to overeat these omega-6 foods.

Unpasteurized, full-fat dairy

Does dairy strike you as a potentially problematic food? I wouldn't be surprised if it did. It is fairly common for Americans today to understand that dairy falls in the questionable category. The most common trope I hear is that dairy is bad because no other animal species consumes milk after infancy.

This is true. Humans are the only species that continues to consume milk after infancy. Does this mean we shouldn't consume milk or other dairy products? Maybe. As with the rest of the conclusions I draw in this book, evolutionary history is an important resource to turn to, but it isn't the final arbiter. We can't rule out dairy products unless there is hard science to back up that decision.

It turns out that there is, but only to an extent. Dairy can fit into both the "to avoid" list and the "to eat" list. It's complicated. Your ability to tolerate dairy could be practically zero, or it could be 100 percent. In general, the bulk of dairy's health problems come from dairy's sugars and proteins, which can be seriously inflammatory. Varieties of dairy that contain sugar and protein, such as milk, yogurt, and cheese, have much greater potential to interfere with health than varieties that are pure fat, such as butter and heavy cream.

All of which is to say that dairy is worth some experimentation. Many women (myself included) experience greater hormonal stability, clearer skin, lighter periods, easier weight loss, and greater digestive comfort when they avoid dairy. I highly recommend eliminating it to see if doing so boosts your well-being. Listed on the following pages are all the important things to bear in mind about dairy and your body so that you can make the best decision for you.

Dairy considerations:

○ **All dairy products have a hormone influence.** Dairy products are some of the most hormonal foods. Because milk comes out of cows' mammary glands, progesterone, estrogen, testosterone, and many other hormones are naturally present in it. Women who are sensitive to hormone fluctuations, particularly those who wrestle with acne, may benefit from limiting dairy products.

○ **The lactose in milk, yogurt, and some cheeses can cause discomfort.** Lactose is the most famous dairy "problem." Many people lose the ability to digest lactose after infancy. Lactose is a sugar that, when not properly digested, can lead to digestive discomfort, bloating, overgrowth of bad bacteria, and SIBO. It's not an enormous health concern, but it is definitely worth consideration for the sake of digestive comfort.

○ **Milk and whey-based cheeses (such as ricotta and brown cheeses) cause a high insulin response.** Designed to grow newborn infants, milk is full of compounds that promote rapid growth. This is great for infants, but it can be problematic for fully formed human beings. Whey protein in particular contains insulin-like compounds that drive insulin levels even higher than plain sugar does.

○ **Milk, yogurt, and cheese can lead to histamine reactions and gut problems.** Next to whey, the other dominant dairy protein is casein. Casein causes two primary problems: 1) It can elicit an immune response called a histamine reaction. Histamines may be familiar to you since over-the-counter medications for swelling and allergies are antihistamines. Histamine reactions can cause acne, skin conditions such as rashes, asthma, allergies, congestion, and other sinus problems. 2) Casein can affect the gut in the same way that gluten and other wheat proteins do, particularly in people who already have damaged guts or autoimmune conditions. Eliminating milk, yogurt, and cheese from the diet can therefore be a key component of healing for anyone with questionable gut health or systemic inflammation.

○ **Pure-fat dairy such as heavy cream, butter, and ghee contains only trace amounts of whey and casein, rendering it easier to digest and less threatening to a sensitive gut.** Milk, cheese, and yogurt contain to varying degrees casein and whey, which can cause unpleasant effects in the body. Since cream and butter are almost 100 percent fat, they do not contain whey and casein and are therefore quite safe. For people who are highly sensitive to whey and casein, however, such as those with leaky gut, "almost 100 percent" might not be safe enough. This is where ghee enters the picture. Ghee is a special, boiled form of butter that has been purified of any residual proteins left in butter. You can find it at most supermarkets or make it yourself at home. (Now, for the most wary, ghee *still* is not guaranteed safe, but it is almost a universally safe bet.)

Beyond being safe sources of fat in the diet, dairy fats are on the "must eat" list for many women because dairy fat is a rich source of vitamins A and D. Moreover, if you can get your hands on dairy products from grass-fed cows, you will benefit from two rare nutrients, conjugated linoleic acid and vitamin K_2. Conjugated linoleic acid may reduce tumor growth, improve immune function, and help with both diabetes and weight maintenance. K_2 is necessary for a wide array of cellular functions, including supporting healthy skin. Many savvy health advocates consume grass-fed butter or ghee specifically to get a daily dose of K_2.

○ **Products from industrially raised cows have a low nutritional value.** Most dairy products that you can buy from a supermarket come from cows raised on corn, soy, and scrap feed in industrial dairy-processing plants. The quality of an animal's diet has a significant effect on its ability to deliver healthful products. Products from cows that were raised in a pasture eating grass (called *pasture-raised* or *grass-fed*) contain a higher percentage of healthy fats (such as omega-3 versus omega-6), higher amounts of antioxidants, and more of precious vitamins like A and E.

o **Low-fat dairy products add sugar.** Mainstream nutrition-ism says that low-fat dairy is healthier than full-fat dairy. This is patently false. Stripping dairy of its natural fats means that other substances need to be added to give it texture and make it palatable. Sugar is one of these sneaky devils. Other processing chemicals follow. There is always a trade-off between fat and sugar in low-fat products. The *Sexy by Nature* diet is not interested in being low-fat. It is only interested in high-quality foods. Full-fat dairy is the most healthful kind.

o **Unprocessed, fermented dairy products can be help-ful for your gut if dairy proteins are not an issue for you.** Yogurt and kefir are fermented dairy products, which means that bacteria is available to you when you eat them. This has two primary implications for your health: 1) the fermentation process breaks down lactose and a significant portion of the pro-teins casein and whey, rendering the products more healthful for digestion and hormonal response, and 2) the bacteria in these products can help replenish and promote good bacteria popula-tions in your gut.

The dairy takeaway

Dairy is complicated. In its typical processed forms, it can damage the gut, hormone balance, and the immune system and can cause weight gain. In its more natural forms, these problems are less significant, and dairy might be well tolerated.

The fattier the dairy source, the less potential it has to cause problems. Heavy cream, butter, and ghee from natural sources are supremely healthful sources of fat for the majority of people.

How to Eat

In the quest for good health and radiant sex appeal, the simple act of eating the right foods is at least 75 percent of the journey. Food is the real deal—it's the stuff of which your DNA is made. Good food provides your body with all the right stuff it needs to *do* all the right stuff, and that makes all the difference. Good food is going to get you leaps and bounds beyond wherever you are now and catapult you into real health, real energy, and real sex appeal. All you have to do is eat the right foods. Eat the right foods. That's it! It really is that simple.

But there is a *bit* more to it. *How* should you eat them? In what amounts, and at what times? These important questions are addressed in detail below. Nonetheless, healthy eating remains quite straightforward and boils down to this simple summary:

> ***Eat sufficient protein, fill in the rest with carbohydrates and fat, don't snack much, don't starve yourself, and develop a healthy relationship with food and with yourself.***

Eat in meals; don't graze

Nutritionists today are obsessed with the idea of eating several small meals a day. This is ridiculous. Sure, you can do so if you want to, and in some circumstances it is important to eat continuously throughout the day, but that's where the good reasoning ends.

The reason medical professionals advocate small meals is that people often experience blood sugar swings that make them cranky, tired, sluggish, and light-headed. The idea is to consume sugar and other foods regularly enough to keep blood sugar levels stable.

What these professionals fail to account for is that blood sugar levels would never spike or plummet in the first place if we ate healthy foods. Blood sugar levels spike only when you consume a lot of sugar, and they plummet only when your body has to exert metabolic effort to keep those high levels in check. Even dense sources of carbohydrates are perfectly well tolerated when they have natural safeguards such as starch, vitamins, and fiber in place.

Eating a healthy diet that keeps blood sugar relatively low removes the "necessity" of eating every couple of hours. Eating in square meals actively *promotes* metabolic wellness. Why? Because every time you eat, you force your body to process food, even if it hasn't finished processing all the food that's already in there. When you eat continuously throughout the day, your body never gets to burn through all the food that gets backlogged. When you eat in square meals, however, it does. Waiting until you are hungry before you eat enables your body to metabolize all the energy left over in your cells.

Eating meals also enables your body to restore proper hunger signaling. If you eat constantly, your body stops understanding what it feels like to be hungry. The signal to eat gets lost in the noise of "Sure, I could eat," and the signal to stop eating gets lost in the noise of "But am I full yet?" Being partially satiated all the time means that your body stops knowing the difference between full satiation and no satiation. This partly explains why snackers need to snack. They just don't have the proper hunger signals flowing through their veins, and they get caught up in feeling both moderately hungry and moderately full at the same time. If it sounds exhausting, that's because it is.

So don't graze. Don't snack (often). Don't eat "six small meals throughout the day." Eat in meals—maybe three a day, maybe four, with a snack here or there. You don't have to be militant about it, but do pay attention. Your waistline, your energy level, your mood balance, your happiness, and everyone you spend time with will thank you.

Eat sufficient protein

It is important to eat sufficient protein each day in order to live, have energy, and achieve mental clarity. Protein comprises not just your muscles, which require protein for maintenance and regeneration, but also your neurotransmitters, which are important for mental well-being, stability, and the ability to fall asleep at night. Protein also has highly satiating effects, so it helps people with cravings regulate hunger signals and stop being hungry all the time. Eating a diet adequate or higher in protein has been shown to be one of the best strategies for losing weight.

Aim to eat between 50 and 100 grams of protein each day. How much is 50 to 100 grams? It's hard to tell without looking at food labels. One very rough estimate equates 100 grams of protein with 1 pound of protein. The more fat a protein source has, however, the more that fat is going to make up a part of the weight calculation. So a 1-pound steak with lots of fat on it has maybe 0.8 pounds of protein, whereas 1 pound of 99 percent lean turkey has approximately 0.99 pounds of protein.

Another good approximation is a can of tuna. One can contains around 25 grams of protein, so imagine eating three tuna can–sized portions of protein every day.

It is important to spread your protein somewhat evenly throughout the day, or to have at least a little with each meal. The more protein you have with each meal, the more steadily your body can process and use that protein for metabolic function. This is helpful for mental clarity, sleep, and energy. It helps keep you satiated and makes each meal a hearty one that satisfies you.

Nuts and seeds contain some protein, but they also come with downsides: a high caloric load, a lot of omega-6 fat, the potential for the fat to be rancidized and therefore highly toxic, estrogenic compounds, and a high phytonutrient (anti-nutrient) load. Animal protein is the best source because it lacks those downsides and is the most complete and vitamin-rich protein out there.

Eat sufficient fat

Eating fat makes us fat, they say. Eating fat gives us heart disease. Eating fat makes us die sooner. None of these statements hold weight when evaluated against rigorous scientific standards.

The problem with fat, much as with carbohydrates, is that researchers—and the media who write about their findings—sometimes fail to distinguish between different kinds of fat. They often study and write about Fat with a capital F and lump all the kinds of fat together in their statements. There are many different kinds of fat, however, of varying quality. To that end, it's important to be specific about the kind of fat we're talking about and its specific effects. In short:

o Omega-6 fats such as seed oils are inflammatory in high doses.

o Deep-frying omega-6 fats rancidizes them and causes oxidative damage.

o Trans fats are toxic.

These are the bad fats. As for the good fats:

o Saturated fat found in animal products is perfectly, neutrally healthful.

o Medium-chain saturated fatty acids such as coconut oil increase energy efficiency and weight loss.

o Monosaturated fats such as olive oil and avocados are uniquely associated with lower mortality risks.

○ Omega-3 fat is anti-inflammatory and reduces both mental and physical health risks.

Not all fats are created equal. Making sure to get enough of the good ones is *crucial* for weight loss, mental health, and metabolic fitness.

Getting enough fat is crucial—but how much is enough?
"Enough" means

1. Eating a fatty fish like salmon one to three times a week to get sufficient omega-3s (unless you take a fish oil or cod liver oil supplement).

2. Eating some fat with every meal to increase nutrient absorption. The more fat you eat with your meals, the more of the crucial fat-soluble vitamins A, D, E, and K (and just about every other nutrient) you absorb. Additionally, the more fat in your diet, the more robust your hormone production will be. Without fat, hormones aren't built properly, and reproductive glands, stress glands, and thyroid glands all suffer.

*Eat a **minimum** of 50 grams of fat per day.
This is the equivalent of one tablespoon of your
favorite oil or half an avocado at each meal.*

The Standard American Diet fears fat because of all foods, fat contains the most calories per gram. This makes it the most energy dense. But is that a good reason to fear fat? It is not. In fact, many people on high-fat, low-carbohydrate diets start eating fewer calories—without even trying!—because they find fat and protein to be so satiating. If you've heard of Atkins, and you've heard that Atkins is a "miracle diet" for some, this is why. Fat triggers the release of "I'm satiated!" hormones and helps the body keep insulin levels low.

Moreover, carbohydrates promote blood sugar fluctuations, which often create an illusion of hunger in the middle of crazed mood swings. Fat by itself does not raise blood sugar levels *at all*. Consuming fat is almost like a metabolic free pass. Best of all is that eating fat in conjunction with carbohydrates slows the release of sugar into the bloodstream, keeping your blood sugar levels much lower than they would be otherwise. Chronically high blood sugar levels are generally not good for you, particularly if you are overweight or potentially insulin resistant. Paired with fat, however, carbohydrates become less problematic. Fat is the hero in this story, and its unique ability to soothe cravings, promote satiation and metabolic fitness, and keep blood sugar levels stable makes it powerfully fat-burning, powerfully health-producing, and powerfully sexy.

> Fat's unique ability to soothe cravings, promote satiation and metabolic fitness, and keep blood sugar levels stable makes it powerfully fat-burning, powerfully health-producing, and powerfully sexy.

Fat also is the stuff of which cellular membranes and many other important molecules are made. With sufficient fat, your tissues become flexible, smooth, and well-coordinated machines. The best and most exciting way you'd probably notice this effect is in the quality of your skin. With an unhealthy-fat or low-fat diet, skin often becomes pasty, brittle, and dry. With a higher-fat diet, especially one rich in ghee, butter, coconut products, and monosaturated fats such as avocados or olives, skin becomes dewy, soft, and smooth.

All of which is to say that healthy fats

o should *not* be feared.

o do *not* make you fat.

o reduce cravings.

o provide unique nourishment.

o promote healthy hormone production.

o promote mental health and stability.

o keep blood sugar levels stable.

○ reduce the risk of Alzheimer's (coconut), improve mental health more effectively than SSRIs and antidepressants (omega-3 fat from fish), and lower your risk of heart disease and stroke (monosaturated fat).

So *eat* it. Nothing to fear here!

Eat an appropriate amount of carbohydrate

Just because fat is far healthier for you than standard wisdom would have you believe does not mean that you need to eliminate carbohydrates. It is true that a low-carbohydrate diet can be uniquely helpful in losing weight, overcoming insulin resistance, and managing diabetes and other noncommunicable diseases, but if you are not wrestling with those conditions and you want to eat carbs, then go ahead and eat them. Just make sure to focus on the sexifying natural ones: vegetables, starches, and fruit.

When to limit carbohydrate intake
One result of the SAD is being overweight. Being overweight is a *symptom* of metabolic brokenness more so than it is a *cause.* How do you overcome it, then? How do you fix the metabolic derangement? How do you start burning fat rather than storing fat? There isn't a magic bullet, but for many people, a low-carbohydrate diet comes close.

Plenty of studies demonstrate that lower-carbohydrate diets improve insulin sensitivity and weight loss for many women. For this reason, if you are overweight, especially if you have weight around your abdomen (which is uniquely associated with insulin dysfunction) or are diabetic or insulin resistant, you may want to consider limiting your carbohydrate intake.

A therapeutic, lower-carbohydrate diet contains around 100 grams or

A therapeutic, lower-carbohydrate diet contains around 100 grams or less of natural carbohydrate per day.

less of natural carbohydrate per day, primarily from vegetables and a moderate amount of fruits and/or starches. Is lower always better? No. The sweet spot is different for every woman. Some women find that limiting carbohydrates too much leads to fat *gain* because it triggers starvation-type responses in the body such as decreased thyroid activity. For this reason, 100 grams a day— which is approximately four pieces of fruit, or two when coupled with a daily dose of vegetables—is an excellent starting point for any woman interested in boosting the efficiency of her insulin response.

When to eat sufficient carbohydrate

Since limiting carbohydrates has been shown to be helpful for insulin resistance and weight loss, many people have thrown the baby out with the bathwater and avoid carbohydrates with un-reasonable fear. Carbs should not be actively feared for several reasons, however.

First, at least half of the people who have succeeded on low-carbohydrate diets and most of those who have been studied are men. This is important because low-carbohydrate diets pose no inherent risk to men. Women, on the other hand, especially those who are not overweight, often require carbohy-drates in order to 1) get the "fed" signal from a more sensitive reproductive system, 2) provide sufficient energy to offspring, and 3) support healthy thyroid function. Without at least some carbo-hydrate in the diet—say, 100 grams a day—many women expe-rience metabolic dysfunction, mood swings, poor sleep, anxiety, obsessive thoughts about food, lethargy, and the wide variety of medical complications that come from hypothyroidism.

Carbohydrates play as much of a role in telling the body that it has been fed as fat does. If carbohydrates are significantly lim-ited, a woman's body can start enacting starvation responses. It might slow the metabolism; it might increase cravings; it might cause insomnia; and it might cause something I call a "fast-ing high," which increases her energy and alertness (not unlike caffeine does) in order to encourage her to spend more time foraging for food. So while a lot of success with low-carbohydrate diets has occurred in both sexes—trust me when I say that they have been helpful for many women, too—the fact remains that a low-carbohydrate diet may push some women over the edge from "adequately supplied with energy" to "inadequately."

It makes sense, then, that women at healthy weights, underweight women, and especially athletes are at the greatest risk for complications with low-carbohydrate diets. These women are more susceptible to running low on energy and causing their bodies to enact starvation responses. Carbohydrates are particularly crucial for athletes since they support muscle function and energetic output. Women who are at least slightly active should eat a few servings of carbohydrate every day.

Many women anecdotally report better moods with carbohydrate intake. Carbohydrates have been implicated in the production of serotonin. This is largely why eating sugary foods feels so good. When you consume a high-carb meal, serotonin, dopamine, and other feel-good neurochemicals spike in your bloodstream. This may seem like a good idea, but the spike doesn't last long,

Macronutrient summary: What to do with protein, fat, and carbohydrate

Once you have sufficient protein in your diet and eat it with most meals, make sure that you also eat fat and some carbohydrate with every meal, then fill in the rest with however much fat or carbohydrate is right for you.

In fact, as long as you are not deliberately restricting carbohydrates in order to pursue weight loss or insulin-sensitizing goals, I encourage you not to pay all that much attention to how much fat and carbohydrate you eat. Rather—and this should come as no surprise—you really should focus on the quality of your food. Eat good carbs. Eat good fats. And everything else should healthfully and happily fall in line.

and sugar spikes come with lots of negative health consequences. Eating natural carbohydrates with meals, however, can significantly contribute to feelings of calm and wellness and even help you sleep better at night.

Regardless of whether you follow a low- or moderate-carbohydrate diet, you should pay close attention to the state of your body. Are you losing weight if you want to? Are you feeling good both physically and mentally? How much carbohydrate works for you is different than it is for other women, and it will probably vary at different points in your life. Experiment to find what works best. Watch and listen to your body, and adjust your eating accordingly.

Break free from the breakfast norm

When confronted with the list of foods I regularly eat, people often gasp: "But what do you eat for breakfast?"

"Food!" I snark back.

American culture is obsessed with sweet, "gentle" breakfasts such as cereal, bagels, pancakes, and toast, with eggs, bacon, and sausage squeezing in under the bar as exceptions. Why, I have no idea. The best answer I can come up with is that we have programmed ourselves not just psychologically but also physiologically to crave carbohydrates in the morning. This is how it works: if you consistently eat the same flavors at the same time, you body becomes adjusted to them and even begins demanding them at that time every day. This is especially true of sweets, and especially true if you are on the standard American blood sugar roller coaster. Low blood sugar when you wake up in the morning makes you need sugar almost immediately in order to feel better.

This is not the best habit. Fortunately, it can easily be overcome.

Breaking out of the sweet breakfast rut requires a bit of deliberate change. For a few days, challenge yourself to eat eggs, bacon, steak, fruit, sweet potatoes, or ideally a mix of all those things for breakfast. Why eat sweets for breakfast? I have no idea.

Why not eat vegetables? Why not just eat the healthiest foods you can imagine at every meal?

I eat vegetables and meat for breakfast every day, and I couldn't be happier. I'm not saying you have to. Maybe you decide to have fruit with breakfast. I do that often. The point here is to integrate fat, protein, and carbohydrates into each of your meals. And then experiment from there, eating the healthiest diet possible that is attuned to your own psychological and physiological needs.

Once you challenge the breakfast norm for a few days, your hormonal needs will begin to shift. Your body will no longer expect you to give it carbohydrates at that time. It will, instead, allow you to feed it what it truly needs and nourish it with wholesome, natural, energy-promoting foods that can propel you through the day. It has been definitively shown that high-protein breakfasts lead to greater energy and higher metabolic rates as well as decreased food cravings throughout the day. Protein in the morning is excellent for your health.

Resist social pressures

I could write a whole book (and indeed many people have) on the variety of social situations we find ourselves in that make us eat foods we don't want to eat. Donuts in the kitchen at work, bagels at the morning meeting, snacks at the bar, potato chips your husband keeps in the pantry, snacks you are supposed to bring to PTA meetings and soccer games...these occurrences add up in a big way. Food—especially unhealthy food—has become integral to the fabric of our daily lives.

It used to be that when people had a treat—a real treat—it was something homemade, rare, and usually on a holiday that was revered because it was the one time a family would come together, give thanks, and feast. But the game has changed. We are now confronted with unhealthy free food several times every day. We are even obligated to participate. God forbid you ever send a child to school without the requisite Valentine's Day sweets.

Be your own ally

Every day we find ourselves socially obligated to be around unhealthy foods, prepare them, and/or eat them. The thing is, you just don't have to. It requires some willpower, but that can be mitigated with finesse and humor. To stay true to healthy foods, my most powerful and helpful motivator is the fact that I actively *want* to be healthy. Once I came to love my own choices and to honestly want to stay away from the foods that were pushed on me, I lost the guilt and shame I had associated with saying no.

When you really believe in nourishing yourself above all else, saying no to food pressure becomes much easier. So how do you do it? You work on it slowly over time. You continue to cultivate your relationship with healthy foods, and you come to love them more and more. You experience the awesome effects of your new diet, and you start to believe in it so much that the external stuff does not matter as much anymore.

Loving your own foods and choices means that you shed the desire to conform to social pressures over time. The point is to arrive at a place where you *choose* to say no to unhealthy foods rather than *force* yourself to say no. Forcing yourself to do things is never pleasant. But when you *choose* health and *choose* love, it stops being about rules and starts being about empowered living.

Say no

Don't let people begging you to indulge make you eat something toxic. They may sincerely have your best interests at heart, but if they love and respect you, they have to let you make the choices you believe are the healthiest for you.

The best way to stick up for yourself is to be firm, loving, and apologetic at the same time. If possible, let your hosts know beforehand that you are okay with bringing your own foods and dishes, or negotiate a meal that is simple and easy for everyone.

Be open about your needs, but don't flaunt them, and don't force your choices on anyone else. You can be healthy, grateful, and a good guest or participant all at the same time. It only requires honesty, sincerity, and open, accommodating communication about your needs.

A quick word on lunch, work, and travel

Pressures arise in the workplace, particularly around lunchtime. I recommend that you arm yourself with your own foods at the office. Keep a stock of almonds, dried fruit, or jerky in your desk. Pack your own lunch. And when you go out, learn which restaurants make dishes that you are happy to eat, or learn how to specify what you want. For example, you can ask for a dish to be prepared in olive oil rather than vegetable oil. Or get a salad with oil and vinegar dressing. It takes some experimentation, but you will learn how to be true to yourself and to enjoy a delectable meal out at the same time.

When you travel, be smart and pack accordingly! If you are going on a long flight, some jerky, fruit, nuts, and avocados will go a long way. Cans of salmon and other fish are also great, and if you're a careful packer, even hard-boiled eggs and veggies can survive the trip. It may take more planning than grabbing something at Cinnabon before you board, but it is always worth it.

Do not restrict yourself

Of all the topics in this book, this is the one I have written about the most. I have written about it until my eyes popped out of my head and my face turned blue, and I imagine this will continue to happen for quite some time. I am glad to do it. The message needs to be spread far and wide, and farther and wider. It really is that important.

***Restriction inevitably leads to unhappy thoughts
and unhealthy behaviors.***

Here's the problem: on a daily basis, women e-mail me and ask me how to stop overeating. I always respond by telling them that they are approaching it from the wrong angle. You can't stop overeating *first*. You need to stop restricting first. **Restriction leads to overeating.** If you restrict yourself, your body will demand that you eat more the next time. You can't stop it, really. And it's not your fault. It's natural. You just need to acknowledge that the more restricted you are and the more deprived you feel, the more you are going to eat in the long run.

Restriction is *bad*. Depriving yourself and stressing out about how much you are eating can get you into a messy relationship with food in a hurry. Restriction makes you dream about food, eat unhealthy foods, and develop bad eating habits that get tied up in your happiness in a nasty way.

What do I mean when I say "restriction"? It varies for many women. Usually it means monitoring calories and deliberately trying to undereat, something most of us have suffered at some point in our lives. I have found that the simple act of writing off specific foods can be equally problematic. Did you swear off sugar? Did you forbid yourself to eat out at restaurants? Did you eliminate dairy even though you don't appear to suffer significant negative health consequences from eating in it?

Writing foods off can be awesome and liberating, but only if you do so as an act of joy rather than an act of restriction or punishment. You may want to try it. It has worked for me in many instances. I simply *cannot* eat dairy products, so I don't feel sad or deprived when I have to pass them up. Yet for those of us who have touchy relationships with deprivation, writing foods off has the potential to make us obsess over them. If this is a problem for you, be flexible. *Don't write things off. Don't be militant.* Your body can handle certain things. You can eat outside your norms from time to time.

And in all cases, you have forgiveness and a powerful body on your side. You can always recover. You can *always* get back on

> Love yourself, forgive yourself, and focus on certain foods because you made the *choice*, not the *rule*.

track. You can always love yourself, forgive yourself, and focus on certain foods because you made a *choice,* not a *rule.*

I know I said that you need to stick to your guns. You do. But don't be your own drill sergeant if it's killing you. Life is about being happy, not about being perfect.

Throw calorie counting out the window

The Standard American Diet lives and dies by the idea that counting calories is the surefire way to lose weight and be healthy. Yeah, calories are important to bear in mind. But do we really need to keep beating this dead horse, especially when a whole lot else is going on?

Calories matter. But two facts of diet make calories *secondary to quality:*

1. Eating a natural, healthful diet of whole foods reduces cravings and makes you eat less—and happily so! Proper hormone balance realigns hunger signaling. You will eat less because your metabolism is no longer broken, and you will do so without feeling deprived.

2. Eating a diet rich in nutrients promotes a healthy metabolism. When you have enough B vitamins, iodine, selenium, copper, zinc, magnesium, manganese, iron, vitamin A, vitamin C, vitamin D, vitamin E, and vitamin K, for example, your metabolism runs without being tripped up by nutrient deficiencies. One of the biggest problems with the nutrient-poor Standard American Diet is that deficiencies in certain nutrients can cause whole organ systems to fail. And if one system fails, then others become hindered. The brain can't

work without a healthy gut. The reproductive system can't work without a healthy thyroid gland. None of these things can work if the molecules from which they are constructed are lacking crucial nutrients.

As metabolic health improves, the body gets better at dealing with shock. It can handle insulin. It can handle carbohydrates. It can handle a night without sleep here and there. It runs faster, stronger, better. It can even handle it when you eat more calories.

Think again of the Big Bad Wolf. It's pretty easy to blow down a house made of straw. But how easy is it to blow down a house made of bricks? How easy is it to blow down a woman's body if it's built from the most healthful, natural, life-giving, and nourishing foods?

It is not easy at all.

Fixing your metabolism helps your body naturally do what it needs to do for healing. This means that it will likely lose weight. Does reasonably restricting calories speed up weight loss? Yes, at least in the short term. Is it necessary, though? No. Is it optimal? I don't think so. What's optimal is nourishment. What's optimal is health. With those two things, weight loss follows. You will eat less. You will give your body the kind of food it needs to lose weight. You don't need to count calories. You simply listen to your body and give it what it's asking for.

Playing nice with your body means that your body will play nice back.

Don't medicate with food; journey beyond emotional eating

I cannot state with more passion and conviction that the *Sexy by Nature* diet promotes mental health and stability, specifically with respect to food cravings. However, you might have a history with food that has disrupted your ability to eat intuitively.

Serotonin, dopamine, and food cravings

Two neurotransmitters in the body need to be properly balanced and present in high enough levels in order for you to have a healthy psychological relationship with food: serotonin and dopamine. Serotonin and dopamine have precursors, which are molecules that the body uses to synthesize them. Many people have found that taking the precursors 5-HTP (for serotonin) and L-tyrosine (for dopamine) drastically reduces food cravings.

Before embarking on this kind of treatment, it is best to consult a healthcare practitioner. Serotonin and dopamine need to be balanced in the body, so it is often wise to get those levels tested before supplementing. If you are interested in pursuing this kind of supplementation, check out *The Mood Cure*, an excellent book by Julia Ross.

Like millions of other women, including me, you might have developed an emotional attachment to food that turns food into medication.

For so many women, we eat when we are stressed, when we are depressed, when we are anxious, and even when we are happy. This is still an issue for me when I spend time with a particular person from my past. It used to be that every time I talked to him, before I even noticed, my hands would have gone in and out of the refrigerator and pulled out a pie tray. *What?* These days, I tend to notice my reaction before I get to the fridge as opposed to after the pie tray is empty. The fact remains, however, that the stress of this situation always sends me right to the refrigerator.

Food is an escape, a distraction, and a means to forget what is going on in our minds and in the world around us. It has a real power to function like a drug, every bit as much as cigarettes, marijuana, and cocaine do. It may be chemically much different from those other substances, but many researchers have proposed that overcoming certain drug addictions is not as difficult as overcoming food addiction. Food is a particularly hard medication to get over because you can never go off of it cold turkey. It is always present in your life. You *have* to eat, and that makes working through emotional attachments to food all the more challenging.

* * *

The way to get over emotional attachments to food, depending on the severity, is different for every woman. I recommend getting professional help or attending Overeaters Anonymous meetings if you struggle in any significant way. You may want to consider psychiatric help for your cravings or natural alternatives of supplementation with the amino acids 5-HTP and L-tyrosine that can promote serotonin and dopamine secretion, thus reducing cravings. Additionally, and perhaps most importantly, we all can benefit from approaching food with awareness and love—more on that in Step 5.

Develop a healthy relationship with your body and yourself

One of the primary reasons women today have disordered relationships with food is that we have unhealthy relationships with ourselves. The vast majority of us are unhappy with our bodies. Some studies report that up to 80 percent of us feel this way.[17] That is not a number to take lightly. Can body negativity be good for our psychological or physiological health? Not by a long shot.

Having a negative relationship with your body means failing to love it. It means not accepting your body for what it is, and wishing your body were different. The same goes for our whole selves. When we fail to accept and embrace ourselves as we truly are, we stop being wholly loving. We become negative. We hate. We nitpick. We loathe. We feel sad and angry.

Why is this bad?

Aside from making us unhappy, it's bad because it sends us into unhealthy eating patterns. As I have mentioned, many of us have negative feelings about ourselves, and we eat in order to make ourselves feel better. But doing so brings about feelings of guilt and shame, which can make us feel worse and make us eat even more. This vicious cycle is almost impossible to get out of without the tools of acceptance, forgiveness, and love on your side. It took me several years.

Having a negative body image and a negative self-image is one of the most destructive things we can do to ourselves as women, both as individuals and as a community seeking empowerment. It is not natural. It should not be normal. It is a painful reality that has been thrust on us as a result of a history of sexism, cultural norms, magazine covers, celebrity worship, billboards, commercials, and the fashion and cosmetics industries. It literally takes lives. It is not necessary, however. It. Is. Not. Necessary.

In fact, this kind of self-doubt is not only unnecessary, but totally possible to overcome once you put the right psychological pieces into play. You *can* triumph over it. Step 5 is all about that. How do you relate to yourself? How do you treat your body? How do you develop psychological habits that promote self-confidence, get rid of negative self-talk, and help you love your body? Are these ideas a pipe dream? Are they really possible? They are. With the simple act of picking up this book, you have already begun.

3: Live

> *"In a massive, long-term study of 17,000 civil servants, an almost unbelievable conclusion emerged: the status of a person's job was more likely to predict their likelihood of a heart attack than obesity, smoking or high blood pressure."*
>
> —MATT RIDLEY,
> *Genome: The Autobiography of a Species in 23 Chapters*

If you have read Step 2 and have started eating the right foods, you've already won the major battle. Your body needs the right nutrients to do its job, and every drop of nutrition you give it makes you a healthier and sexier woman. Welcome to the club—the *Sexy by Nature* diet is the sexiest diet in the history of humankind.

Welcome to the club— the *Sexy by Nature* diet is the sexiest diet in the history of humankind.

But there is obviously more to it. Just as ancestral women ate vegetables, game, organ meats, and natural fruits instead of chips, crackers, bread, and soda, they also slept for significant amounts of time, lived by natural lighting, and relaxed instead of pulling all-nighters or working 60 hours a week in a fluorescent-lit cubicle. To which I can only say: "It sounds too good to be true!"

Nonetheless, we *can* live in harmony with our bodies, even in the modern world. It's not a fantasy. Sure, we're not cave dwellers, and we don't read by firelight, and we don't spend all day outside in the sun. But here in the industrialized world, we have the incredible luxury to prioritize our lives the way we want to, more or less. We can get plenty of sleep every night. We can minimize harsh lighting, especially in the evening hours. We can spend time in the sun (or at least supplement with vitamin D). We can exercise in a way that benefits our bodies. And we can have values that make our lives meaningful. It's about knowing what is good for you as an independent, natural woman and *choosing* to have those things in your life every single day.

Stress

Stress is a demand made on your mind and body—a call to action. This call has real physiological effects; stress has the potential to be monumentally harmful. Of all the lifestyle components discussed in this book and in other health books, stress receives the most emphasis, and with excellent reason. Stress has been linked to depression, anxiety, early death, poor immune function, illness, inflammation, and just about every noncommunicable disease, including diabetes, heart disease, cancer, obesity, and autoimmunity.

Cortisol: The stress hormone

When you encounter a stressor, your body's main reaction is to secrete cortisol. Cortisol's job is twofold: it wakes you up and primes you for activity on one hand and decreases the functions of "unnecessary" body systems such as digestion, reproduction, and the immune response on the other. Elevated levels of cortisol in the blood are associated with:

○ alertness, which makes it a challenge to fall and stay asleep

○ decreased immune system power and efficiency

○ increased blood pressure

○ weakened connective tissue in the organs and skin, which creates premature wrinkles

○ sugar being released from the liver, which increases blood sugar and insulin levels and decreases insulin sensitivity

○ leaky gut

○ inflammation

○ elevated levels of male sex hormones in the blood

○ decreased fertility

○ disrupted sleep patterns

Stress and digestion

The stress response shuts off bodily functions that are not necessary for immediate survival. Your adrenal glands, which are responsible for directing the stress response, believe that your energy is better directed toward survival.

Ever experience digestive distress when you are worried? Go a whole week without a bowel movement because you're in a new place? Or get diarrhea or gas before a big event? These issues arise largely because of the stress response. Your gut is intimately tied to your mental health and your state of stress. In moments of high stress, your bowels may tighten or loosen to extreme degrees that cause instantaneous seizure or release, leading to prolonged constipation or immediate mortification. Worse is the long-term effect of stress on your gut. The more stress you experience, the more your gut flora take a hit and your intestinal walls can become inflamed. Stress contributes to leaky gut in unhealthy and difficult-to-control ways.

Stress and your ovaries

Perhaps even more striking is the impact of stress on reproduction: a significant number of women experience infertility based solely on stress at some point in their lives. This is true of primates as well. Apes at all levels of the social hierarchy eat the same diet, but those at the bottom of the ladder have irregular menstrual cycles while their more popular and relaxed peers do not.

Stress tells the body that it's not a good time to reproduce or even to expend energy on reproductive function. When you are stressed out, your pituitary gland can't pump out a robust supply of hormones with any semblance of regular timing. Under stress, the pituitary gland fires in fits and starts, and hormone levels decline more and more over time if you continue to bear the same load of stress.

This is one of the primary facts of life that makes women's health so different, more complicated, and perhaps even more delicate than men's health. The reproductive system is inordinately sensitive to stress, perhaps more so than any other system in the body. Fertility, sex drive, skin health, and mental health are all at stake in the battle between stressed and relaxed states in your body.

Inflammation, stress, and why you get sick under pressure

Just as the stress response turns off digestion and reproduction, it also turns off (in a rather complex fashion) the immune response. At some point in your life you may have gotten sick *after* a big event. This is because, just like with digestion and reproduction, stress puts the immune response on hold. If it hadn't been on hold, you might have been able to respond appropriately at the time and avoid getting sick. But because you were unable to mount a defense against the illness when your body needed it, the illness was able to work its way in under the radar. When your body finally picked up on the signal, you had a nastier and more widespread problem to deal with, and your immune system overcompensated with vigorous, panicked action.

Stress has immediate, small-scale effects on colds, flus, indigestion, and the like. It also has the longer-range and more powerful effect of inhibiting your immune system's ability to fight off cancer, heart disease, autoimmune disease, and other long-term

Caffeine and your adrenal glands

I don't expressly forbid caffeine in this book. In all fairness, caffeine has been used therapeutically for many conditions. But if you are under stress, sleep poorly, or experience impaired hormone status of any kind, ditching caffeine should be a serious consideration.

Caffeine promotes alertness in two primary ways. First, it blocks the activity of certain chemicals in the brain that help you achieve drowsiness. Second, it increases neuron firing, which accounts in part for why your mind might race or you might experience anxiety while on caffeine. In response to hyperactive neurons, your adrenal glands produce adrenaline and cortisol, which makes your heart beat faster, tenses your muscles, releases sugar into your bloodstream for extra energy, increases your blood pressure, and decreases blood flow to your extremities.

damage. Your immune system takes care of you in a wide variety of serious ways. If you turn off your immune system, you may be opening yourself up to big-time problems.

Stress from an evolutionary perspective

Comparing modern humans to ancestral humans demonstrates why stress is such a big deal. In ancient humans, the stress response worked as it was intended to. Stressors such as hunting prey, being chased by predators, and other such escapades were immediate events that required high levels of energy, focus, and bodily response. When a lion came into camp, for example, the stress response leapt into gear to do its job. Adrenaline flooded the system, and the stress hormone cortisol shut down all nonessential bodily functions temporarily. This enabled our ancestors to become hyper-alert and energetic and devote all their resources to the task at hand: survival. A sleepy hunter-gatherer was a dead hunter-gatherer, at least where lions were concerned.

Today, we work 40, 50, 60, 70, or 80 hours a week. We stay up late at night. We drink espresso. We have kids with soccer practices and homework assignments and college loans. We have breakups and loneliness and low self-esteem. We have mortgage payments and taxes, a terrifyingly corrupt political establishment, and weapons of mass destruction. We have, perhaps worst of all, a constant barrage of media that reminds us of how endangered we are on a daily basis. Stress is pervasive in our lives.

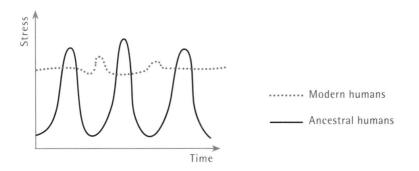

The fact that modern stress operates as a moderate thrum rather than periodic spikes means that we run constantly on cortisol. Digestive, reproductive, and immune systems falter. Skin acts up. Sleep is disturbed. We rarely get the chance to relax properly. If the body doesn't calm down, it doesn't get a chance to heal or to breathe. It is always running, always trying to catch up, always creating fires faster than it can put them out.

I think the real story is a bit more complicated than this picture, though. Was it all about lions and running and high-stress events for our ancestors? I don't think so. I don't think the graph is as perfect as I have drawn it. Ancestral humans probably had relationship trouble. They probably fought over friends and politics and cultural norms, which I'm sure they had plenty of, too. They probably worried about the weather, the upcoming hunting season, and the integrity of their shelters. So stress is not wholly abnormal. It's okay to have stress. It's natural. It's just not natural to have so much of it and never to relax.

Minimizing stress

With all this knowledge about how stress can negatively affect your health, the name of the game is minimization. It would be impossible to live a stress-free life. It might even be boring. Without stress, there would be no challenges, no true emotional depth, no journeys, and no transformation. Stress is an integral part of life, and it's okay to let it run its course.

You need to work with your body. All unnecessary stress in your life should go. There's no reason for it. Even stressors that may seem unavoidable are in fact perfectly avoidable. Do you really need to participate in PTA meetings? Do you have to enroll your children in four different after-school programs? Must you apply for that promotion at work? Why?

"Why?" is the most important question to ask about stress in your life. Why are you doing a particular thing? If the answer is not strict necessity or desperate wanting, and if the activity is causing you emotional upset or putting undue demands on you and your body, let it go. Reconceptualizing and reprioritizing are the only ways to overcome stress.

Take a promotion at work, for example. Sure, the extra workload may increase your salary or your prestige. But do you need a higher salary? You might not. Do you need prestige? Not really. How do those two things compare to family, friends, love, laughter, and leisure? They might not be worth it in the end. It's hard to let go of some things, but making small changes over time teaches us that *nothing* is more important than being at peace with our bodies and ourselves.

Some stressors are even harder to let go of because they are deeply woven into the fabric of our brains. Many women are perfectionists, for example. That's pretty stressful. In fact, for some women, it's downright debilitating. Perfectionism can cause infertility. It can decimate libido. It can make it impossible to sleep.

How do you stop being a perfectionist? Lots and lots of practice. Lots and lots of therapy. Lots of good friends and self-love and self-care. Patience and forgiveness for yourself as you trip up and move forward. Focusing on the things that bring you wellness and peace rather than validation and fear. If you orient your life toward harsh standards and perfectionism, you are going to run yourself into the ground. The trick, then, is to forestall it by removing perfectionist-type stressors from your life.

Anything that gives you worry, anxiety, or mental anguish is a stressor. Insisting that you are not good enough, feeling pressure to perform or to be special, fearing certain situations...these are powerful causes of stress that have the power to kill you. Literally.

Stress and magnesium

One of the most powerful physical things you can do to support your body in times of stress is to supplement with magnesium.

Magnesium is one of the most abundant minerals in the body, second only to calcium. It plays a crucial role in more than 300 enzyme reactions. It is essential for the manufacture of ATP—the primary energy molecule in the body—as well as for the proper contraction of heart muscles and blood flow. It also helps your body calm down after a stressful event. Without magnesium, your muscles, nerves, and neurons would be incapable of shutting off.

One of magnesium's roles is to open channels on the walls of your cells. When your body needs you to respond to a stressor, magnesium opens the channels and calcium floods into the cells. The calcium helps your cells rev up and be active, and then magnesium opens the channels again to pull the calcium out of the cells. With insufficient magnesium, calcium has a hard time leaving the cells.

This is important for stress because calcium in brain cells keeps them firing and calcium in muscle cells keeps them tense. In essence, the presence of calcium causes you to remain continually stressed. You have a hard time letting go of thoughts. You experience anxiety. Your whole body becomes a tension-filled mess. Magnesium helps relax you. It is crucial for recovering from stressful events.

Unfortunately, magnesium isn't found in foods today in the quantities it was throughout human history. It used to be ubiquitous in water and in the soil, but factory farming has stripped the environment of much of its magnesium. There are few dietary sources apart from greens, legumes, seaweed, and chocolate. For this reason, a magnesium supplement is in order for just about everybody. The recommended daily dose for women is 400 milligrams. I take between 300 and 700 milligrams, depending on how much stress I am under. Magnesium glycinate is a form of magnesium that is gentle on the gut, is easy to absorb, and can be found in any grocery store.

An Epsom salt bath is also an excellent way to get magnesium. Soak in a full bathtub with two cups of Epsom salts for thirty minutes, and you'll feel loose, relaxed, and more peaceful.

What to do about it:
tips for the chronically stressed

○ Make an agreement with your family or housemates that you will receive a certain amount of "me time" every day.

○ Do your best to sleep for as long as possible.

○ Allow yourself to nap during the day if you feel the need to.

○ Create a safe space in your home that is yours alone.

○ Keep your environment clean and organized.

○ Take a few minutes every evening to stretch, meditate, and breathe.

o Develop a quick morning or evening routine that centers you around what really matters.

o Keep a list someplace visible—such as on your mirror—of all the things that are truly important in your life: family, friends, love, charity, faith, God, community, and harmony are all good examples.

o Carry with you or wear a piece of jewelry that centers you around these important things.

o Develop networks of support.

o Think deeply about what you need to feel peaceful, safe, and happy. Create a list, and work on integrating those things more fully into your life.

o Have conversations with your loved ones about your needs and how everyone can work together to meet them in balance with their own.

o Smile, even when you don't feel like it.

o Practice saying no when a proposed activity exceeds your ability to feel safe and peaceful.

o Consider therapy to help you prioritize and reclaim your mental balance.

Sleep

When was the last time you consistently got seven to nine hours of restful sleep? Did it last for a whole week, or several weeks, or even years? Is it not the most magnificent feeling in the world to wake up naturally, without an alarm clock, feeling rested, alert, and ready to face the day? To go to sleep easily and wake up a whole, fierce woman who is capable of anything?

Messing with sleep is a powerful stressor. The problems caused by poor sleep are nearly identical to the problems caused by stress. Without proper sleep, the body secretes stress hormones to perform the important function of keeping you awake. This is perfectly healthy on a day-to-day basis—you do need to be awake sometimes, after all. But when you miss out on sleep, your body secretes inordinate amounts of stress hormone to make up for it. It also ends up secreting stress hormones at the wrong times—for example, late at night rather than in the morning. If you go out partying until 4 a.m., your body is going to pump cortisol into your bloodstream during a period in which you would ordinarily be asleep. Then you experience a disruption in your circadian rhythm, which can be quite harmful for the regulation of organ function throughout your body.

There are many different theories about the kinds and amounts of sleep that are natural for human beings. For example, some experts think that ancient humans slept whenever it was dark outside. Others think that ancient humans slept in two distinct chunks during the night with a period of wakefulness in between. Others think that we need regular catnaps during the

Humans are designed to get a lot more sleep than we do today.

day. But there is one major point of consensus: humans are designed to get a lot more sleep than we do today.

What good sleep looks like

As far as sleep scientists can tell, the most restful and healthy sleep:

○ **Contains at least four, if not six, REM cycles.** REM stands for rapid eye movement and characterizes the phase of sleep in which the eyes move back and forth quickly. REM cycles are important for processing the events of the previous day and committing new facts to memory. Alternating with REM cycles are periods of deep sleep that are also crucial for wellness.

○ **Is long and deep enough for optimal hormone production.** Sleep is the most powerful period of the day for hormone production.

○ **Occurs in a completely dark room.** Melatonin, the hormone primarily responsible for putting you to sleep, is poorly secreted when exposed to light. Darkness helps your body put you to sleep.

○ **Is not artificially interrupted.** Interrupting sleep disrupts the repair processes that occur during deep sleep.

○ **Is emerged from naturally, without the aid of an alarm clock.** Waking on your own means that you have gotten all the rest you need.

Benefits of good sleep include:

○ Feeling good, rested, and alive

○ Rapid healing of skin, acne, and scar tissue

○ Improved memory and recall

○ Faster recovery from exercise

○ Decreased allergic response

○ Decreased systemic inflammation

○ Better decision-making

○ Better mood

○ Reduced irritability

○ More rapid cellular and bodily detoxification

○ Optimal immune system recovery and function

○ Healthy sex hormone production and increased libido

○ Reduced cravings

○ Increased muscle growth from growth hormone secretion

○ Decreases in and prevention of tumor growth

Health risks of poor sleep include:

○ **Decreased leptin sensitivity.** Leptin is the hormone responsible for controlling food intake. If you are leptin insensitive, your food cravings can run out of control, tricking you into thinking that you are hungrier than you really are. In particular, leptin insensitivity can cause sugar cravings, weight gain, diabetes, and obesity.

○ **Decreased insulin sensitivity.** Insulin resistance shows up immediately after one night of decreased rest, and one week of sleep deprivation results in a diabetic insulin profile. Repeated abuses inevitably lead to a weakened insulin response.

○ **Weight gain.** Largely due to increased cravings, decreased insulin sensitivity, and stress hormone secretion throughout the day, poor sleep may be one of the driving reasons behind America's obesity problem.

○ **Decreased female sex hormone output.** The female sex hormones estrogen and progesterone are produced during sleep. So are LH and FSH, hormones from the pituitary gland that tell the reproductive organs what to do and play crucial roles in menstruation. With impaired sleep comes impaired estrogen, progesterone, and LH and FSH signaling, as well as dysregulation of the menstrual cycle and all sex hormone production.

o **Decreased antibody formation.** The immune system recharges and creates antibodies at night. Without a sufficient supply of antibodies, your body is more susceptible to illness.

o **Impaired memory.** Short-term memories are stored and cemented overnight. Have a big test or presentation in the morning? It's probably better to sleep on the information you've already learned than to cram all night, or you may not be able to remember anything come test or presentation time.

o **Depletion of magnesium stores.** Magnesium is crucial for good rest and recovery from stress, as well as for energy production and hormone function.

o **Shortened telomeres.** Telomeres are crucial for a long life. Shortened telomeres are a mark of premature aging and are statistically correlated with higher risks of high blood pressure, stroke, and heart attack.

o **Increased skin and organ aging.** Without sufficient time to repair tissue damage overnight, skin and organs accrue successive damage and become damaged and dysfunctional sooner.

What to do about it:
sleep hacks for experts and insomniacs alike

Some people have a natural knack for sleep. I definitely do not. I have been an insomniac my entire life, although recently my sleep has improved significantly. Here are the best ways to improve the quality and duration of your sleep naturally:

o Supplement with 400 to 600 milligrams of magnesium a day.

o Consider herbal remedies. I have seen passionflower work well for many women. Chamomile, mint, and other teas are quite restful and promote sleepiness.

o Consume protein consistently throughout the day to support optimal neurotransmitter and particularly melatonin production.

o Reduce sugar consumption to maintain consistent blood sugar levels. If blood sugar fluctuates to a significant degree, adrenaline can wake you in the middle of the night. The body often secretes adrenaline in response to blood sugar lows.

o While reducing sugar consumption, keep healthful, natural carbohydrates in your diet. A carbohydrate-rich meal approximately four hours before bedtime can promote the production of serotonin and other molecules that help you sleep.

o Sleep in a completely dark room to support melatonin production.

o Expose yourself to the blue light of the sky (or fluorescent light) during daytime hours. This is the opposite side of the coin to darkness and melatonin production. Being awake during the day helps your body know when to go to sleep at night.

o Limit exposure to artificial light, and particularly fluorescent or blue-tinted light, after sunset. This point is crucial for many people. Put lampshades on your bright or blue-tinted lights, experiment with candlelight, and keep lights dim later at night. Your body will not produce melatonin in the presence of blue light.

o Decrease exposure to TVs and other screens before bed.

o If you use a computer, download free f.lux or similar software (justgetflux.com). This software automatically changes the tint on your computer to orange based on when the sun rises and sets in your location. f.lux nearly saved my life.

o Turn down the brightness on your screens.

o Make sure that your sleeping space makes you feel safe, comfortable, and at home.

o Do not exercise before bed; do it earlier in the day.

o Consider standing at your desk, which can help your body feel awake during daylight hours (and therefore sleepy during nighttime hours).

Standing

A quick Internet search on the phrase "how many Americans sit at work" yields a fascinating, if frightening, field of articles. Today it showed me, in this order: "Sitting at Work: Why It's Dangerous and What You Can Do" *(The Huffington Post)*, "Sitting for Hours Can Shave Years Off Your Life" (CNN), "Are We Sitting Ourselves to Death?" (MedHelp), "Obesity expert says daily workouts can't undo damage done from sitting all day" (NBC), and "Can Sitting Too Much Kill You?" *(Scientific American)*. Clearly there's something going on with sitting, and it's so obvious and important that just about every online news source has covered it.

These days, we sit a lot. Studies have shown that upwards of 35 percent of American adults—approximately 50 million people—are completely sedentary.[18] They sit still at their jobs, have no regular physical activity or exercise regimen, and are inactive around the house. Even more Americans live on a threshold just above that, managing to get some activity and participate in some sports, but still sitting for a continuous eight hours a day at work. Most nine-to-five jobs require sitting, and therefore most of us sit all day every day without fail.

Research has suggested that sitting is one of the worst factors affecting American health. A study conducted by the American Cancer Society found that women who sat for more than six hours a day were about 40 percent more likely to die during the course of the study than those who sat for fewer than three hours a day. Other studies have shown that these women have a significantly increased risk for cardiovascular disease, obesity, type 2 diabetes, and depression. In one study, those who worked a sedentary job demonstrated almost twice the risk of a specific type of colon cancer.[19]

Worse, we are not doing anything effective to counteract this problem. Exercise does almost *nothing* to reverse the effects of excessive sitting. Adding leisure and athletic activities on top of a mostly sedentary day does not reduce the risk of these diseases.

How metabolisms get lazy

In one model advocated by obesity expert Dr. James Levine, the metabolism is like a fire that requires stoking. Even an hour or two of hardcore cardio exercise once a day cannot undo the damage done by sitting all day. The more you sit, the slower your metabolism gets. Your muscles stop moving, and your heart slows. This makes sense from an evolutionary perspective. The human body burns fewer calories at rest, and as it detects less and less of a need to burn calories, it sinks further into metabolic sluggishness. Insulin effectiveness drops, and the risk of developing diabetes and heart disease increases. This results not just in decreased metabolic rates and efficiency but also in lethargy, brain fog, and the need for an afternoon nap.

Most people who use standing desks report increased alertness throughout the day. Their bodies do not shut off the way they might if they were sitting. Standing has been one of the greatest boons to my own writing career. I used to fall asleep at my desk all the time. These days, I never feel too tired to work.

What's more, standing, walking, and moving slowly throughout the day have eclipsed exercise as my favorite and most efficient ways to stay in shape. Instead of working my body into the ground, I simply opt to walk to work, and I exercise only as a leisure activity. My weight seems much easier to manage, and I do not fight abdominal fat the way I used to when I worked out hard several days a week.

What to do about it: move, move, move!

The best non-dietary step to take for good health and metabolic fitness is to break the tyranny that sitting has over your life.

There are two primary ways to do so. The first is to start standing. Just stand. See what happens. Buy yourself a fancy standing desk if you like, pester your employer to buy one for you, or construct a standing desk of your own by piling boxes or large books on top of your normal desk (this is my method). It may be uncomfortable at first, but only because it is unfamiliar. I have never spoken with someone who tried standing at work and disliked it.

My personal experience has been truly transformative. I used to get horrible headaches while working, and I felt fatigued and nodded off to sleep without being able to stop myself. Now, I feel alert, I get more work done, I have energy while I work, and I generally enjoy my work a whole lot more. Now that I have made the switch, I can actively feel my body slowing down, getting tired, and shutting off when I sit. When I stand, however, I feel the blood pumping energetically through my veins.

The other solution is to break up periods of sedentariness with movement. Since your metabolism registers states of rest while you sit, getting up and moving around once every thirty or sixty minutes jump-starts it. Ten minutes of walking every hour should do the trick. I usually go for a quick walk around the perimeter of the building I'm in. Other times I go into an empty room and do squats. This is not the most elegant solution, but it gets the job done and helps me feel awake again. Taking the stairs at work, commuting to work on foot, integrating a walking or biking routine into your life, or doing more physical labor around the house are other great ways to keep your metabolism running good and hard throughout the day.

Sprinting

When health and weight loss come up in conversation, exercise is inevitably one of the first remedies suggested. "Eat less, exercise more," everyone says. Is eating less and exercising more really the key to health? Exercise is important, granted, but not the punitive, excessive type of exercise so often practiced in our culture. The *Sexy by Nature* approach to exercise focuses instead on happy movement, and supplements that with sprinting and weight-bearing exercise tailored to your own goals and needs.

The highest priority: happy movement

Exercise deserves to be a high priority in your life, but it should come easily, healthfully, and in a variety of forms. Yes, you should exercise. But should you drag yourself to the gym for spinning class at 5:00 every morning? Not unless you want to collapse in a heap of wrecked organs in a couple of years. Exercise is good. Too much exercise is bad.

To be a long-term solution, the type of exercise you do should make you happy. If you're engaged in an exercise that doesn't increase your love of life or facilitate a harmonious relationship with your body, throw it out the window. It's not doing you or your body any good. Trust me when I say that there is a type of movement out there that will bring you

> If you're engaged in an exercise that doesn't increase your love of life or facilitate a harmonious relationship with your body, throw it out the window.

joy. Find movement that you do because you *love* it, not because you *have* to do it. It will make all the difference in the world.

Options for happy exercise include dancing, swimming, cycling, gymnastics, yoga, Pilates, Zumba, aerobics, Frisbee, martial arts, and all sorts of team sports. Even yard work will get your heart pumping. Activities that prioritize enjoyment over calorie-burning are best. For example, dancing is monumentally better for me than working at an elliptical machine. Why? On an elliptical, all I'm trying to do is burn calories, or perhaps get better at climbing stairs. Dancing, however, is first about feeling embodied and alive and interacting with other people and only secondly about burning calories and building muscle. Movement that makes you happy is not an act of force, but an act of love.

> Movement that makes you happy is not an act of force, but an act of love.

Bird-watching is a great way to log miles while focusing on something else. Geocaching is another fun way to get out and about. What better way to exercise than to go on an adventure seeking buried treasure? If being outside makes you happy, try to integrate more walking into your daily routine. Love the mall? Go window shopping on a weekly basis. If you haven't yet found your happy exercise, rest assured that it is out there. Try the classes at a local YMCA, gym, or university. Check out meetup.com for groups of people who are doing a type of exercise that you think you might like. Groups are powerful motivators. Nothing helps you enjoy exercise more than doing it with a friend. Friends take your mind off of what might be difficult and help you focus on having fun instead. This is what life is all about, right?

The most beneficial type of exercise: sprinting

If you are driven by fitness and weight-loss goals, you may want to expand your exercise regimen beyond happy movement and into the realm of training. What kind of exercise gives you the

> ## Maximum heart rate
>
> Calculate your maximum heart rate by subtracting your age from 220. The sweet spot for fat-burning, according to conventional wisdom, is 60–70 percent of that number. Most typical cardio training happens at 70–85 percent of maximum heart rate, where you are breathing heavily for an extended period. Above 85 percent is the *anaerobic threshold,* or the sprinting area. At this point, you should be sweating and gulping air. The anaerobic range is where HIIT exercise occurs.

greatest health benefits and the most weight loss? Sprinting does. Not *running;* sprinting. There is a difference. When you run, you jog along at a consistent pace. When you sprint, you move as fast as you can for a short period of time.

One of the catchphrases for sprint-based exercise is "high-intensity interval training," or HIIT. Instead of spending hours doing cardio—whether it's running, biking, or slumping over an elliptical machine—in HIIT you spend short amounts of time working at a higher intensity. Doing so has enormous health benefits relative to traditional cardio training and takes a fraction of the time.

Traditional cardio training is inferior to sprinting in that:

○ **It can increase oxidative stress and damage,** which leads to aging and illness.

○ **It can depress the immune system,** largely by raising cortisol levels and inflaming the body.

○ **It has lower metabolic and fat-burning potential,** at least relative to HIIT. Overweight people are told time and again that in order to lose weight, they just have to start running. This could not be further from the truth. Cardio exercise can be actively harmful for health and weight-loss goals, depending on your hormonal status and your physical health. Fat metabolism may decrease with cardio exercise because cardio exercise elevates cortisol levels, which can impair insulin sensitivity. It can also decrease fat-burning by convincing your body that it is starving. If you live in a calorie deficit because your exercise level is too high, and especially if you are stressed out on top of that, your body may respond by down-regulating thyroid activity. The more you run, the slower your thyroid production might get. Thyroid hormone is crucial for high metabolic rates and an efficient metabolism.

○ **It is often antagonistic to weight loss.** Studies have shown that most people end up eating more to make up for the calories they burn in cardio training. In fact, doing thirty minutes of cardio may be better for weight loss than doing sixty minutes of cardio.[20] The real benefit of exercise comes from moving *at all* rather than reaching a specific duration.

○ **It can be antagonistic to heart health.** Studies of marathoners have found higher rates of cardiac events in marathoners than in non-marathoners. In one study, one in ten marathon finishers had elevated scarring on heart tissue.[21] (Other studies have shown that the damage is temporary.) Marathoners are of course healthier and live longer than couch potatoes, but this kind of exercise has long been touted as being the pinnacle of health, which is obviously not the case.

○ **It does not promote muscle growth.** Marathoners are good cases to highlight here as well. Picture an Olympic marathoner. She's thin, right? Super-thin? Maybe even with baggy skin? Compare that image to the physique of a sprinter. Sprinters are muscular, fit, and vibrant. High levels of cardio exercise can force the body to metabolize protein in the body rather than fat, especially if fat stores have been significantly burned through.

As harmful as chronic cardio may sound, movement is still important. Any kind of exercise is quite good for you. Exercise conveys benefits for cardiovascular health, diabetes risk, and weight loss. Cardio is just not the best. Sprinting is better because it burns fat, enhances the flexibility of arteries, decreases the risk of heart disease, and sensitizes the body to insulin. The benefit comes largely from the fact that sprinting reduces the amount of time the body spends in stress mode—and therefore reduces the stress response—while maximizing the muscle and strength-building capacities of your workout. All from approximately 20 percent of the time investment.

Specific health benefits of sprinting/HIIT:

○ Improved blood cholesterol profiles

○ Decreased blood pressure

○ Increased oxygen use by muscles

○ Removal of metabolic waste from muscles during resting periods

○ Increased insulin sensitivity

○ Increased resting metabolic rate

○ Reduced risk of stroke, acute coronary syndrome, and overall cardiovascular mortality[22]

○ Increased time available for relaxation, fun, sex—whatever you like!

Sprinting and happiness

Sprinting also happens to be excellent for increasing the amount of endorphins, serotonin, and dopamine in your body, which give you a natural happiness high. Once I get going in a sprint workout, I often find it challenging to stop. This is why exercise is as effective at mitigating depression as antidepressants and is one of the most important lifestyle factors to add to a depressed patient's regimen.[23]

What to do about it: go real fast!

High-intensity interval training can come in the form of running, biking, rowing, doing push-ups or squats or burpees, or any other exercise that makes your heart beat so fast that it feels like it's going to leap out of your chest. Most studies demonstrate that the health benefits of HIIT come from at least thirty seconds of going as fast as you can.

So you sprint really fast for a short period, and then you rest. You perform this cycle again in a little while, and you keep rehashing it until you feel like you've gotten a good amount of exercise. Don't overdo it—just a few cycles can be an excellent workout for women who have yet to get into the groove.

The thing about exercise is that it varies for every individual. I cannot give you hard-and-fast numbers to stick with. I can, however, provide estimates. As a beginner, fifteen to thirty seconds of running or biking as fast as you can followed by two minutes of rest is a probably good place to start. Run until you need to stop. Your body will tell you when. The important part is to ratchet up to that 85–90 percent of maximum heart rate threshold, and then let it drift back down to a more normal level. Doing so enables your heart to increase its aerobic capacity without undergoing the stress of pumping at an increased rate for hours at a time. Repeat your sprint interval five or six times.

As you progress in your exercise regimen, slowly increase the amount of time you spend sprinting as well as the number of intervals you perform. It should come naturally as you do it more. I recommend sprinting two to four times a week, with four being the upper limit. Over-exercising is not good for a woman's body. Your body needs sufficient recovery time to be assured that it is well fed, in a state of peace, and healthy enough to produce thyroid and reproductive hormones.

Strength

The second form of exercise that's great for your health and your metabolism is weight training. Muscle mass plays a significant role in health and metabolic function. The health benefits of muscles through weight training include:

○ **Removal of glucose from the blood for storage in the muscles as glycogen.** This can prevent advanced glycation end-products from running wild in the bloodstream and damaging organs and tissues.

○ **Increased growth hormone production.** Growth hormone, often called the fountain of youth, is critical for maintaining lean body mass and burning fat. It has also been known to fix DNA damage and to promote healthy growth in children.

○ **Brain growth and repair.** The hormone BDNF, which is stimulated by exercise, helps brain cells regenerate into old age.

○ **Increased basal metabolic rate.** Muscles burn more calories than fat does. When you build more muscle, you burn more fat.

○ **Improved heart health.** Healthy muscle mass, including but not limited to heart muscle, enables the heart to pump more effectively, which reduces blood pressure.

○ **Protection of joints and bones.** Having more muscle means that you rely less on your joints to move around, which protects your back, ankles, knees, and hips.

○ **Increased bone strength and density.** Weight-bearing exercises increase your body's fortification of bone reserves. Strong muscles also protect your skeletal frame. This is particularly important for women given the risk of osteoporosis.

o **Increased longevity.** Muscle mass has long been associated with longer life. As people age and the amount of exercise they do decreases, muscle tends to waste away, being metabolized by the body after years of disuse.

o **Enhanced strength and performance.** Muscle growth is phenomenal not just for strength but also for endurance. Weightlifting can create non-bulky muscles that have stronger and stickier fibers, which provide power for all sorts of exercise.

o **Increased insulin sensitivity.** Just as the need for insulin decreases because muscles can store glucose, weight training can increase insulin sensitivity. Increased insulin sensitivity leads to increased fat-burning and a decreased risk of diabetes.

o **A curvaceous body.** Many people believe that curves come from fat. This is true—fat in your breasts, hips, buttocks, and thighs contributes to a sexy figure. However, muscle tone can help turn a woman's hourglass figure into a powerhouse of curves. Muscle tone tightens the stomach, narrows the waist, and shapes the behind and legs in gloriously feminine ways.

Don't be afraid of gaining muscle!

Many women express a fear of becoming bulky when they start lifting weights. This fear is completely ungrounded. Here's why:

Muscle growth occurs largely as a result of male sex hormones, so putting on muscle is quite a bit more difficult for women than it is for men. It is obviously possible for women to put on a lot of muscle—we have all seen female fitness competitions—but it takes diligence and hard work. If you see a woman with veins popping out of her muscles and thighs rippling as she walks, chances are quite good that she spends a *serious* amount of time and energy cultivating those muscles. If you think those muscles are hot and you want them, you can get them by lifting heavy weights for long periods using specific training regimens, which you can read about in a wide variety of weight-training guides. On the other hand, doing push-ups and lifting weights a few times a week will give you a beautiful tone and shape, but never a masculine look. It's impossible for a woman to develop a masculine physique or bulky muscles without deliberately setting out to do so. You don't have to worry about becoming bulky from the exercises recommended in this book—unless you want to be.

If you start strength training and notice new muscle definition (and you likely will), the appropriate response is celebration. Muscles are healthy. They are enormously good for you. They help give you curves and shape. What reason do you have *not* to celebrate? Muscles are *beautiful* for all these reasons.

What to do about it: pick up heavy things

One of the common reasons women avoid weight training is that it's intimidating. If you are one of these women, I don't blame you. Trying to figure out those weight machines at the gym is more than a little off-putting. This is exacerbated by the fact that many gyms are real meat markets, full of men with lots of muscles who may act like they own the place.

My advice to you is this: do not use the machines. They are unnecessary. Machines target one small muscle group at a time and are inferior to free weights and body weight exercises that target several muscle groups at once.

Lift weights, then. Use dumbbells. Pick them up in front of you, to the sides, behind you. Pick up as much weight as you can. The more weight you put on your muscles, the harder they have to work, and the more repair and growth they will do. Even five repetitions of one incredibly difficult movement is enough to make a significant difference. How do you know how many repetitions you should do? Do what feels right. Your muscles should be fatigued at the end. Muscle fatigue is the best measure of all.

Another option is to lift your own body. Do push-ups of all different kinds. Keep your knees on the ground if that's easier for you. Put your hands under your shoulders and lift yourself off the ground, keeping your body as straight as possible. Turn over, sit on your butt with your feet out in front of you and your arms behind you, and lower yourself to the ground. Doing both front-facing and back-facing push-ups works an enormous range of muscles in your arms, and you should be toned in no time.

Squats and sit-ups are other great ways to use your own body weight. For a squat, stand with your legs shoulder width or a bit wider apart. Keep your knees pointing forward, and bend your knees until your behind is as low as it can get—hopefully somewhere near your ankles. Then stand. Repeat. Trying doing several dozen or even 100 at once. For a sit-up, lie on the ground with your feet out in front of you. Bend your knees, keeping your feet flat on the ground. Curl your upper body toward your legs. Sit all the way up if you can. If not, come up a bit of the way, and hold it there. By doing a few simple exercises like sit-ups, squats, and push-ups along with some form of sprinting, you will become an exemplar of fitness in no time.

Exercise from an evolutionary perspective

The way we exercise today is pretty far removed from the way people have done it throughout human history, as just about every physical fitness guru will tell you. Exercise used to be a simple fact of life. It came from natural movement—from hunting, from play, from working in the environment. Today we go to the gym and move machines around. It's not natural. But it is often the best we can do, so we need to pay close attention to how we can harmonize our bodies with the methods available to us.

As far as scientists can tell, ancestral humans (and current traditional cultures) spent a fair amount of time walking. They

The dangers of over-training

Exercise is important, but you can overdo it. Unfortunately, millions of women, particularly young women, overdo it every day.

Over-exercising occurs more often in women than it does in men. A woman's body is sensitive to starvation and stress in ways that men's bodies just aren't. The negative effects of over-exercise begin cropping up for women at different points, so I can't tell you outright what the upper limit is for you or anybody else. I can't necessarily prevent you from over-exercising. I can, however, share with you what happens when you over-exercise so that you can recognize the signs.

Over-training causes your stress hormones to fire at a higher rate, which can lead to acne, insomnia, low libido, food cravings, and other hormone malfunctions. Your muscles can't rebuild themselves fast enough, and your body might start burning muscle for fuel. Your joints become fatigued and may become inflamed. Your immune system stops functioning properly, so you may get sick. Your fertility may suffer. Your magnesium stores get used up, which can lead to anxiety, insomnia, depression, and a long list of other disorders.

Over-exercise is a real danger if you work out every day or more than once a day, if you have to make yourself exercise, and if you do cardio or sprint workouts too often. There is a sweet spot for every woman. It may take time to figure out what feels best for your body, but the most important thing to bear in mind is that you must *listen to* and *nourish* your body above all else. Always do what you think is best for your natural body over the long haul. If it wants to rest, let it rest. As you work in greater partnership with your body, you will find that the right amount of exercise comes naturally to you.

engaged in hunting, gathering, erecting shelters, and performing other low-level aerobic activities on a daily basis. We want to mimic these patterns and be moving as much as possible throughout the day.

Ancestral humans also spent time doing serious interval and muscle work. They had to sprint to escape from predators. They had to chop wood or carry heavy loads over long distances. It is obvious that they used their bodies in unique and powerful ways.

All this comes together in a diverse picture. Ancestral humans moved in a bunch of different ways. Certain people were probably more fit than others, just as it is today. Some of us are athletes, and some of us are not. Athletes don't have a monopoly on good health. Those of us who move around at least sometimes, however, do. Those of us who mix up forms of movement and don't over-stress our bodies do even better.

What to do about it:
combine happy movement with strength training and sprinting

The best way to achieve harmony between your physical activity and your natural body is to combine a low-level activity that you love, like dancing, swimming, biking, hiking, or playing Frisbee, with a handful of higher-intensity sprinting and weight-bearing exercises every week. I recommend as much low-level activity as possible (including standing at work or walking or biking to work if you can), with two sprint workouts and one or two weight-training workouts per week. The ideal amount of exercise varies by individual, but this is a good and healthy place to start for anyone looking to optimize free time as well as health benefits.

The most important thing is to meet your body where it is. Give yourself the kind of movement you need. Do not overtax your body, but don't sell yourself short, either. If you are obese, seriously overweight, or ill, start as slowly as you need to. Whatever movement you can do is going to help. Increase it over time. As you gain fitness, you will be able to meet and exceed the recommendations outlined here.

Sex

Eating and sleeping are two of the most basic things we do as living organisms. That's why they take up so much space in this book. But there is one other thing we do that every other organism on Earth does: we make babies.

Pregnancy was the name of the game for ancestral humans. Women spent the majority of their adult lives pregnant. Today, however, we have the enormous privilege of being able to choose (more or less) when we get pregnant. Conceiving and caring for children has become an option rather than a necessity. Birth control is one of the greatest innovations of the twentieth century. Where would feminism be without it? Gender equality would be even harder to achieve than it already is.

Birth control is one significant way in which modernization has altered the sexual landscape, but it is not the only way. Evolutionary biologists and psychologists do not agree about what human sexuality looked like back in the day—theories range from very monogamous to wildly polyamorous—so we do not know for sure how best to meet our bodies' sexual and relational needs. The fact of the matter is that we are evolved bodies living in a modern world, and we must develop our own healthy ways of incorporating natural sex drives and sexual activity into our everyday lives. Sex can be greatly rewarding, both psychologically and physically.

Here are some of the benefits of healthy sex and sexuality:

○ Sex relieves stress and lowers blood pressure.

○ Sex boosts immunity by increasing levels of powerful immune system antibodies.

○ Sex can be a great workout—cardio, strength, or otherwise.

○ Higher rates of sexual activity are correlated with a lower incidence of heart attacks.

○ Sex releases oxytocin, the "cuddle hormone" that facilitates bonding and intimacy between partners.

○ Oxytocin also boosts levels of painkilling endorphins. Pain thresholds are vastly reduced in the wake of sex. Migraine sufferers generally report reduced pain after sex.

○ Coupled with prolactin, which also rises during sex, oxytocin promotes sleep.

○ Orgasms force the uterus to contract, which can help rid the body of cramp-causing compounds, leading to reduced menstrual cramping.

○ Uterine contractions may help blood and tissue to be released more quickly, shortening the duration and severity of menstrual periods.

○ Sex releases hormones such as testosterone and estrogen, which can help pull you out of a hormone deficiency if you have one.

○ Increased estrogen from sex can improve the quality of your skin and hair, as well as provide relief for symptoms of menopause.

What to do about it:
explore according to your own desires

Much as I think sex is one of the most important aspects to take pride and ownership in as a natural and empowered woman, I cannot tell you what to do about it. I can, however, support you in your sexual journey by writing a book about how to be healthy and feel sexy that includes all the different medical and natural ways to practice birth control. Both an extensive list of birth control options and a guide to enhancing your libido can be found in Step 4. These are excellent and practical ways to help you explore your sexual self.

Again, I will make no prescriptions about what kind of sexual behavior you should undertake. Please do what fits best with your personal beliefs and experiences. All I can say definitively is that sexuality is a *right,* and that you have the privilege, power, and worthiness to embrace and explore your sexuality if you so choose. Sexuality is a natural part of who you are as a natural woman, and you have nothing to be ashamed of. To the contrary, standing up for and developing a positive relationship with your sexual self is one of the best things you can do to improve your relationship with your body, your relationship with yourself, and your excitement to be in the skin you're in.

Sunlight

Humans have always lived around trees and in shelters, but our ancestors spent much more time outside than we do today. This is especially troubling for those of us who work indoors and watch the sun climb up into and down out of the sky every day through office windows. Is it natural or healthy for humans to live under fluorescent lights? Are we missing out on something important when we don't spend time in the sun?

When I was in fourth grade, I was asked to write an essay on the sun: is it a friend or a foe? I thought that was the silliest question that could have been asked. Obviously it was a friend! Without the sun, we would not exist.

The question was directed toward the issue of skin cancer. According to the article we read—and to many dozens of articles I have read in recent years—the sun is something to fear. We need protective clothing, glasses, hats, and lotions. Never mind the fact that humans have been living under the sun for millions of years without getting skin cancer. What we need is SPF, and we need it *now*.

There is a grain of truth to this panic. With the release of chemicals called chlorofluorocarbons into the atmosphere several decades ago, the Earth's ozone layer became significantly depleted in areas around the North and South poles. Thankfully, this damage has been halted, but it doesn't change the fact that harmful UV rays that used to be neutralized by the ozone layer now penetrate the atmosphere in pretty large swaths across the globe. Most incidences of skin cancer, however, occur in the general population that lives outside of those immediate ozone danger zones.

What's the deal with skin cancer,
and what does the sun have to do with it?

There is an obvious correlation between skin cancer and sun exposure. People who experience severe sunburns before age 18, for example, have a significantly increased risk of developing skin cancer later in life. However, several other factors complicate the picture and indicate that we may want to spend more time under the sun:

○ Sunburns arise in response to intense sun exposure after a period of no sun exposure. A person with a tan doesn't burn. Only people who regularly hide from the sun experience sunburns. In human history, people regularly spent long periods outdoors. They built up strong skin and had no problem being exposed to the sun. When they started to feel like they were burning, they probably moved out of the sunlight. The feeling of burning is a built-in mechanism designed to protect human health. The next day we can go back into the sun for a longer period, and with more and more exposure we develop our ability to live outside. People today typically don't live this way. In addition to staying indoors all day, we wear copious amounts of sunscreen, which prevents us from building a healthy tan and living naturally under the sun.

○ Skin cancer, like other cancers, arises as a result of DNA mutation and poor immune response to the mutation. The mutation can be triggered by extreme sun exposure. However, cancer is supposed to be manageable for the human immune system. The immune system naturally fights cancer and, if healthy, should be able to fight off many cancers. This fact is somewhat alarming with regard to skin cancer because vitamin D is crucial for immune system function and for fighting cancer, but the body's vitamin D stores are almost entirely reliant on sun exposure absent of SPF.

○ Cancer is an epidemic far bigger than the skin. Just as ancestral humans did not get skin cancer, neither do any other animals.

There is no cancer in the wild—no lung cancer, no prostate cancer, and no skin cancer. Sun exposure does not give other animals cancer, and it shouldn't cause human cancer, either. We get cancer in response to the sun not because the sun is a foe, but because we subject ourselves to sunburns, our bodies are inflamed, and our immune systems are compromised.

Why we need the sun: vitamin D

The most important health benefit of sun exposure is the production of vitamin D. Vitamin D has been shown to be one of the best preventative factors in human health: hundreds of studies link vitamin D deficiency to higher rates of many forms of cancer, as well as heart disease, osteoporosis, multiple sclerosis, and other autoimmune conditions. Vitamin D boosts hormone function and production; it has been shown to help with polycystic ovarian syndrome, one of the primary causes of female infertility; and it is supremely helpful for anxiety, insomnia, and depression. Most importantly, it is crucial for supporting a healthy immune system, which can help with short-term illnesses such as colds and flus as well as long-term battles such as cancer and autoimmune disease. The evidence is clear: we need vitamin D in order to be healthy and happy.

> The evidence is clear: we need vitamin D in order to be healthy and happy.

What to do about it: bask

Exposing your skin to the sun is the best way to get vitamin D. You can get some vitamin D from eating salmon or drinking fortified milk, but that's it as far as food sources go. How much sun exposure should you get, then? Exercise caution. Do *not* burn.

The skinny on skin cancer, SPF, and vitamin D

The problem with sunscreen is that it might prevent sunburn, but it has not been shown to protect against melanoma in any statistically rigorous fashion. Moreover, because sunscreen blocks UVB rays, it also blocks the body's ability to synthesize vitamin D. UVB rays are precisely the rays you need to make vitamin D. You might be protecting yourself from sunburn when you wear SPF, but you are not necessarily protecting yourself against melanoma, nor are you synthesizing vitamin D.

But expose yourself over short periods. Build up a tan as much as you can. Develop a tolerance for the sun, and spend more and more time outside for better vitamin D production as well as tan maintenance.

I recommend 20 minutes of daily exposure sometime between the hours of 10 a.m. and 2 p.m. for starters. Increase the duration as you see fit based on how dark your skin is. People with darker skin absorb less radiation, which protects against cancer, but they also need more time in the sun to benefit from its vitamin D synthesizing properties. The more regular your sun exposure, the better your tolerance will be, and the more vitamin D you will send coursing through your veins to the aid of your immune system.

Sometimes it is simply impossible to get enough sun. Even if you make a significant effort, you might not be able to get what you need. In this case, supplementing with 2,000 to 5,000 IUs of vitamin D a day works quite well. Get your blood tested before you begin a supplementation regimen, however. Your doctor is your best resource for calibrating how much vitamin D is right for you.

Spirit

Much of what I discuss here in Step 3 is about differences between ancestral and modern humans. What were humans built for, and how has the modern world distorted the body's ability to meet those needs? How can we get into greater harmony with our bodies and our genes? These last few sections do not deal explicitly with these differences, at least not on a physical level. However, we have many natural needs that go beyond the physical, and the following are some suggestions for navigating and optimizing a few of them.

Aside from the work I do in women's wellness and nutrition, I am a full-time philosophy student. Most of what I study falls in the realm of spirituality. What are people's ideas of God and the universe, and how do those ideas play into their lives and their wellness? These are my favorite kinds of questions, and they have significantly informed my view of human beings and how we achieve health and happiness.

One of my favorite movements in the philosophy of religion is the idea that humans are *homo religiosus*.[24] Looking back to the earliest available evidence in the realms of human art and intelligence, we find artifacts from religious rites and rituals. People were having funerals long before they were conducting scientific experiments. They also had star charts and carvings of constellations, drawings of animals and spirits, and a reverence for the natural world. For as long as we have been human, we have needed to make sense of the world.

> For as long as we have been human, we have needed to make sense of the world.

Life is big. Life is overwhelming. Life is full of enormous questions that no one has any idea how to answer. Religion is a response to those questions. Philosophy is another response, but of a slightly different flavor. And spirituality is the umbrella under which most of these responses fall. Science has provided us with many answers, but it will never tell us why we are here, what happens to us when we die, or why anything exists in the universe at all. These answers may forever elude us. They may forever reside in the realm of myth, wonder, and mystery.

Spirituality may be particularly powerful for women because it gives us a sense of belonging to a larger whole or of being subsumed in something larger than us. I say that it may be helpful for women in particular due to my experience working with women who struggle with their relationships with food and their bodies. Many of these women cite God or other higher powers as important in the healing of those relationships. With God, they say, they have trust. They do not have all the power or all the answers, but God allows them to trust in the greater flow of the universe. Spirituality helps them stop hanging so desperately onto the edge of life, trying to control everything. It helps them forgive themselves and breathe deeply. It helps them trust the world a little more and learn how to walk with less fear among food, culture, and anything else that makes them feel like less than they truly are. It is particularly powerful, in my observation, when women equate higher powers with love. Doing so enables them to become more self-loving and self-forgiving and to feel more at home in their bodies and in this world.

Is spirituality necessary in order to be healthy? Sexy? Happy? Not at all. You are free to do what makes you feel the happiest and the most at peace. I mention spirituality as a part of the book only because it has been transformative for so many people throughout human history, and frequently for the women with whom I work.

What to do about it: whatever you want!

The Big Questions lie at the heart of much of what we do. How you view the world shapes how you act, how kind or fearful you are, whether you trust other people, and whether you feel at home in nature and in your body. What do you believe in? How do you see yourself fitting into the cosmos? Do you have spiritual practices, and are they grounding for you? You could meditate, read, explore, sing, hike, play music, dance—anything that makes you feel connected, grateful, and alive. You could go to church, do daily readings, participate in small-group spiritual circles, or practice yoga. You could surf the web for a spirituality app for your phone, which could be one of the dozens of meditation apps, yoga apps, apps for pulling up quotes from spiritual and philosophical gurus, or apps for spiritual texts. You could belong to any group or interact with any number of people on this level. Communities are powerful parts of many people's spiritual lives; they help us feel at home in this great, confusing, beautiful mess of a universe.

There are infinite ways to orient yourself to the universe. You don't need to believe in God. You don't need to be a part of a religious community. You don't need anything official. You don't even have to know what you think about any of it. But if you are on the hunt for a centering practice, I recommend looking at your history and the world around you and experimenting with the ideas you have encountered. Consider viewpoints and communities that have been particularly helpful to you. What did you learn at Sunday school or in college or on that enlightening road trip that gave you a sense of wholeness? You might be surprised by the profundity and peace you discover when you move forward with these ideas in your pocket.

Settling

When I hear the term *settling,* I often think of settling down or allowing myself to marry someone I don't like all that much. *Settling* has negative connotations and often implies failure. It implies giving up, letting go of dreams, and letting happiness float away.

I chose the word *settling* for this part of the book mostly because it starts with an S, to be honest. I was excited about all the S words I found for this chapter. Another word for the concept I intend to outline here might be *acceptance.* Settle, accept, breathe, relax. I hope to convince you that settling is a good thing.

For too many reasons to count, our culture is largely built on the idea of *running.* We go everywhere quickly, and we have to achieve everything all at once. A little bit is never enough. We always want more. We need more—more things, more toys, more food, more prestige, more money. We need more houses, more cars, more freedom, more education, more choices. We continually chase after more things, but to what end? Does it make us happy?

My opinion is that more things do not make us happier. Simple living makes us happier. Settling down, accepting what we have, looking around us and smelling the roses...this is the stuff that makes us human. It resonates deeply within our bones. We all know that the rat race doesn't bring genuine happiness. Getting out of the race usually does.

For the first few decades of my life, I ran every place I went. I knew exactly what time it was at any given point in the day, I knew exactly what I needed to get done and in how much time, and I hurried to get those things done. I finally realized that I was a perfectionist. I was chasing success and achievement—but to what end? Was it going to give me happiness, fulfillment, or meaning in my life? No, it wasn't. There was no way it could. So I endeavored to slow down.

These days, I walk almost everywhere, and I refuse to go at a faster pace than what comes naturally to me. It was an adjustment, but I have integrated stillness into my life. I have begun walking more slowly, deliberately smelling the flowers, and taking time every day to settle down. It is one of the most powerful things I have ever done for myself, my spiritual life, and my happiness.

When you stop looking for happiness in the rat race, you can find delight in restfulness. The world becomes a place to savor, a beautiful and lovely place. You have more time for friends. You have more time to be kind. You have less to worry about, with fewer things demanding your time, attention, protection, and money. You move toward a state of floating, relying on the depth of personal interaction, connection, and meaning in your life rather than avoiding those questions by staying so damn busy all the time (or by watching TV or clicking through your Twitter feed). I am not telling you to give away your big-screen TV. What I am saying is that a slower life can be a healthier life.

The stress of choice

Choice is one of the greatest freedoms available to us, and I give thanks for it daily. Choice can be a significant source of stress, however. When you go to the supermarket, for example, you have perhaps 600 different varieties of breakfast cereal to choose from. Fortunately, I have liberated you from that particular choice. No more stressing over which variety of Special K to buy! But what about the rest of the choices you face? You might have eighty varieties of candles to consider. Worse, you might have a choice between a job in Michigan and a job in California, or between two different cars, or between one friend or another. Choices are wonderful—they give us freedom. They also tend to stress us out.

Studies have shown that having more choices doesn't make people happier. Even having more money with which to make those choices doesn't make people happier. Above an annual income of $40,000, which is considered enough to live a middle-class lifestyle, happiness levels off. All we really need to be happy is to have enough to survive without worrying. More money and more things do not make a happier woman. Not at all.

I would argue that having more things makes us *less* happy. It certainly does for me. I make it a rule to own no more than I can fit in my car, aside from furniture. When I begin to exceed this limit, I get nervous. The more stuff you own, the more you have to protect, care for, worry about, and devote mental energy to. We devote so much of our lives to worrying about the things we own. Worse, we live in a constant state of acquiring more things and making more choices about those things. This cycle creates so much pressure! How do you choose the right thing? And once you choose it, how do you protect it? Where do you put it? What do you do with it?

What to do about it: settle, prioritize, and simplify

True happiness comes from mindset, relationships, feeling comfortable in your world, and building a meaningful life. It does not come from the frenetic parts of Western existence—busyness, perfectionism, and the acquisition of stuff. I undertook a strong reshuffling of my priorities and got rid of all the superfluous things in my life. Goodbye, clock radio! Goodbye, garbage bags full of old clothes! Anything that I hadn't used in the last 365 days went out the door. Any activity that wasn't enriching my life or the lives of the people around me got erased from the calendar. Clearing up my life in this way has significantly reduced my stress, given me space to breathe, and given me space to be a woman in greater harmony with the things that matter.

The word *settle* has a lot of important meanings here. It means to simplify your choices and your life. It means to prioritize appropriately. It means to be calm. It means to let the dust settle naturally and let life flow without trying manically to control outcomes or achieve goals. It means finding peace with your body, spirit, and life and accepting things as they are. It doesn't mean giving up on dreams; it means pursuing those dreams mindfully.

Settling also means to breathe deeply, live simply, and let go of consumerism, the rat race, and anything else clouding your mind. This may sound like a radical overhaul. In some ways, it was for me. It happened slowly, and I had complete control over it. I made some changes quickly, while others took me several months or even years (and many others I may never fully achieve). I didn't need *more* to be happy. What I needed was *liberation from more.* I needed to be freed from the rat race and from perfectionism. Look around, breathe deeply, and love what you have. I promise that if you undertake this exercise, it will not turn out badly for you.

Striving

Did I save the best element of living for last? Possibly. Striving is a healthy and awesome balance to the idea of settling.

Just as life can feel empty without slowness, life can feel empty without purpose. Purpose can come in any number of forms: a dream job, a promotion, family, artistic pursuits, volunteering, being a good friend, or advocating for social justice, for example. People find purpose all over the place. It is abundant in the world.

So many people are looking for happiness and fulfillment. Where are *you* going to find it? What gives *your* life meaning?

Having a purpose may be the most crucial component of my wellness. Much as I love and promote the idea of self-love, the most important thing I have done for myself in the last decade or so was to shift my focus away from myself. I needed a larger vision around which to orient my life. My purpose is my career. It is the work I do in health and spirituality and in academia. It is about promoting depth, wellness, and love. Obviously, my own being is still more or less my highest priority; none of us can really escape that reality. But on a day-to-day basis, I do not focus primarily on myself. I do not obsess over cultivating charm, skills, or self-love. I do those things, certainly, but I let my purpose chart the course of my life. It is the center of my concern, and my loyalty to my purpose gives me the greatest sense of worth I have ever experienced.

When you care deeply things, their inherent worth gives *you* inherent worth, which provides a calm center from which you can live your life. That has been my experience, at least, and the experience I have witnessed in working with other women. As much as we look for love and happiness inside ourselves, sometimes we need to be a part of something bigger. That purpose informs our identity and gives us a sense of peace and excitement about being alive.

Purpose doesn't have to be a grand plan. But it is helpful to always be striving and to keep your eyes on the future. Health. Education. Family. Community. Progress. Art. Love. Make yourself better, and make the world better. The more you live this way, the more you will feel at harmony with yourself and feel excited about your role in the world.

What to do about it: do!

"Do not think about what the world needs," says Howard Thurman. "Think about what makes you come alive, and go out and do it. Because what the world needs is people who have come alive."

What do you care about? If you can't think of much, explore different options. Trust me when I tell you that you have passion. What makes your heart sing? What are your most important values? What causes, people, or goals do you think about when you daydream? Something as simple as being a good friend can give you the sense of importance and joy that you need to feel purposeful.

Set goals and work toward them. Keep them vigorously in sight and don't let go (unless you want to!). You don't have to achieve these goals in one day or by means of a straight path. Just have them, and keep your eyes on the prize. Every step is worthy of celebration. Every step makes it apparent how crucial you are to your friends, your goals, your job, or your art. Every day you embrace and live into your purpose is a day to delight in the importance of your existence.

4: Overcome

No body is perfect. That's a fact—perfection is just not possible. Personally, I do not want a perfect body. Why reach for an ideal that is, by definition, unreachable? Why hold myself to an impossible standard? And even if I ever got close to it, would achieving that ideal fulfill me in any real way? I doubt it.

However, it is entirely within the realm of possibility to obliterate obstacles that stand in your way. A perfect body is off the table. A body that is strong and healthy and lovely and vibrant...a body that is no longer hindered by the aches and frustrations brought on by the Standard American Diet...a body rich with confidence and life: *this* is not only possible, it is probable. At your fingertips. In your bones. A body that is sexy by nature is not a perfect machine that fits into molds constructed by magazines, but it is healthy, strong, curvaceous, and fit. In this section, we'll dig into the specifics that make it happen.

So far, we've got food down pat. That has won you the major battle for health and wellness. You've got the lifestyle considerations, too. Now it's time to understand your body more deeply and to attack the specific problems that concern or interest you. Has PMS gotten you down your whole life? Do you struggle with acne? Or do you just want more radiant skin? Do you wish that you understood female weight loss better so you could be less frustrated and more successful in your efforts? Here, we leap headfirst into taking action that heals, optimizes, and sexifies.

Things may not be or end up as perfect as you'd like. Each of us comes with a set of genes and a history that complicate healing. I might not hit upon the right prescription for you. These things take time, patience, and love. And even then you need to be aware

of what is truly within the realm of possibility for you and where
you should rightfully set your expectations.

This chapter is about healing. It's about living. And it's
about becoming intimate with your femininity. Here, you learn
all about what's going on under the hood of your various health
problems and are thus enabled to really listen to, understand,
and harmonize with your body. Take these steps forward with
love and patience, but shoot for the stars and see what happens. It's amazing what the female body can do when properly
nourished.

How to approach this chapter:

1. **Identify the problem you wish to address.**

If you are wrestling with a specific health issue, see your doctor, have tests run, and learn the shape of your problem as best as
you can. The more information you have, the more empowered you
will be to overcome it by taking the most appropriate steps for your
healing.

2. **Acknowledge that all health issues are interrelated.**

Even as you work on your acne, your insomnia, or your diabetes, it's important to know that none of these issues really lives
on its own. The most important thing you can do for yourself is
to eat natural foods. A diet this healing and nourishing is hard
to beat, and it will support your body in ways you never could
have anticipated. As you troubleshoot the issues outlined in this
chapter, set goals in the context of the wider whole. Don't neglect
one part of your health for another. Support your whole body,
listen to your whole body, and let your whole body be your guide.

3. **Troubleshoot.**

As you make changes to your diet and lifestyle, document the
changes you observe in your body over time. As positive change
happens, celebrate. If negative changes occur, back up, think about
what happened, and try something new. Finding what works best

for you takes experimentation. Don't obsess, but don't give up on finding your answers. They're out there. Move forward with patience, excitement, and love.

4. **Work with doctors, nutritionists, functional medicine doctors, and other health professionals who can get to know you and troubleshoot your health with you.**

Seriously. I am a good starting point, but I am not an expert in your body, not by a long shot.

5. **Don't expect perfection, but expect kick-ass results.**

Significantly improving your health problems may be lightning fast, or it may take a long time. It may take effort, patience, and lots of forgiveness for yourself and your body as you move forward. Things will never stop evolving, and life will never stop challenging you with obstacles to overcome. Please do not expect perfection. But expect kick-ass results.

Energy:
Be vibrant

Low energy is one of the most common but most difficult-to-address issues that plague women today. How do you put a diagnosis on the symptom "I feel tired a lot"? It's impossible. There are, however, specific mechanisms in the body that can be optimized for the best possible energy. There are also a handful of specific health issues that can be obstacles to a truly energetic life, which include sleep and circadian rhythm disruption, poor thyroid health, blood sugar regulation problems, and insulin signaling problems.

How it works: poor sleep

It almost goes without saying that poor sleep makes you tired. The kind of sleep that turns the mere need for an occasional nap into full-time fatigue comes in many flavors and for many reasons, though the primary problem is usually not getting a sufficient amount of deep sleep, one of the phases of the REM cycle. At night, the body cycles in and out of REM sleep. Each cycle lasts approximately ninety minutes, and four to six cycles should occur every night.

Each stage of the REM cycle is uniquely restorative, whether by deep relaxation, tissue repair, or memory banking. When you get less than the optimal number of REM cycles, your body feels it. You crave that extra cycle; you need that extra rest. You lose out on REM cycles when you sleep fewer hours than you need—typically seven to nine, though it varies by individual. It also happens when you sleep fitfully or wake often during the night, which can be a result of stress, circadian rhythm disturbance (see below), hormone imbalance—especially estrogen insufficiency, which is why so many menopausal women have trouble sleeping—or a wide variety of sleep disorders, such as narcolepsy and nightmares, which I don't have space to cover in any depth here.

Wakefulness and the adrenal glands

The natural cycle of sleeping and wakefulness is facilitated largely by the adrenal glands. Cortisol, the stress hormone, is the primary means by which you stay awake. This is not a bad thing. When you need to wake up in the morning, your body secretes cortisol. When it's time to go to sleep at night, cortisol should have fallen to its lowest level. There's a natural rhythm to the way the body secretes cortisol throughout the day. It becomes problematic only when you force yourself to be awake longer than your body would like, or when you endure stressors that throw your natural and healthy cortisol function off balance.

Stress causes your body to fire cortisol into your bloodstream no matter what time of day you experience it. In times of crisis, your body goes into states of hyper-awakeness and hyper-alertness that generate even more cortisol, which can keep you up late at night, wake you in the middle of the night, or force you to wake too early in the morning. Decreasing stress throughout your life—not just in the hours before you go to sleep—is crucial for keeping cortisol levels low, for keeping your body on track with the natural flux of your circadian rhythm, and for getting a good night's rest.

How it works: the circadian rhythm

Circadian rhythm refers to the natural cycling of time in a human life. Your circadian rhythm—often called your biological clock—accounts for when you wake up, when you feel alert, and when you go to sleep. The more established and healthy your circadian rhythm is, the more robust, regular, and intuitive your sleep and wake cycles are. Your circadian rhythm is monitored by enormously complex machinery that exists in each of your cells. If this rhythm becomes irregular for any reason, it's nearly impossible to feel perfectly alive and energetic throughout the day.

Naturally, a body wakes around dawn. Blue light—the color of daylight—is one of the primary triggers for wakefulness, so your body naturally begins to stir when the sun rises. This wakefulness trigger is detected primarily by the eyes, which makes sense—that's where the light comes through most of the time. However, sensors are present in your skin cells as well. When you are in a space lit by blue light, your body automatically switches into higher gear. For a healthy individual in a healthy setting with natural lighting, then, waking up is a breeze. You'll have slept a full night, gotten all your REM cycles in, and been woken by your adrenals in sync with your body's natural rhythm and the rising of the sun.

The primary ways in which you can disrupt your circadian rhythm are:

O Forcing yourself to stay up too late

O Waking too early

O Waking with an alarm clock

O Not getting enough sleep

O Experiencing stressful events, particularly late in the day

O Eating in irregular patterns, which can surprise your body

O Exposing yourself to blue light when you shouldn't (such as by viewing computer screens late at night)

What to do for circadian rhythm disruption:

O Expose yourself to blue light from the sky (the best source), sunlight-mimicking lamps, or fluorescent light during daylight hours.

O Minimize exposure to blue light in the evening by switching to orange-tinted bulbs and candlelight. Orange light is gentle on the eyes and skin and will not cause wakefulness. There are free programs for the computer that note the time, track local sunup and sundown hours, and change the tint of the screen from blue to orange to match the pattern of the sun. I mentioned the program f.lux in Step 3.

○ Go to bed and wake up at the same times every day.

○ Reduce stress as much as possible, particularly in the evening hours. It's crucial that your stress hormones have time to filter out of your blood and for the glands that produce them to relax as you wind down. The general guideline is that it takes ninety minutes for adrenaline to significantly work its way out of your blood.

○ Get off coffee. Some people drink coffee without problems, but if you're a poor sleeper, eliminating coffee is a good solution to try. Coffee actively increases adrenal activity. Even if you drink coffee only in the morning, the fake energy it gives you can be enough to throw off your ability to calm down the rest of the day. And if you drink coffee throughout the day, your adrenals fire more and more, and their effects are felt later and later in the day.

○ Chocolate and teas that are not labeled "caffeine free" or "herbal infusion" are also caffeinated; try limiting them as well.

○ See Step 3 for more general sleep recommendations.

How it works:
hypothyroidism and the thyroid gland

A slow or malfunctioning thyroid gland is one of the most commonly investigated and diagnosed problems in modern women. If you haven't suspected your own thyroid gland, chances are good that you know other women who have. And rightfully so: the thyroid gland is crucial not only for energy, but also for weight management, metabolic function, reproductive health, clear skin, immune function, and just about everything else. Men have thyroid glands, too, and they can experience hypothyroidism, but they do so at rates far lower than women, largely because they lack the complex relationship between female hormones and metabolic health.

Because the thyroid gland is responsible for cellular energy, it makes sense that when the thyroid gland stops working properly, your energy can get zapped.

The nuts and bolts of thyroid hormone production

Thyroid function is often difficult to optimize because the thyroid gland is intimately connected to other glands in the body. It resides in a chemical cluster of several different glands: the hypothalamus, which is the ultimate hormonal command center, the pituitary (reproductive) gland, the adrenal (stress) glands, and itself, the thyroid (energy) gland.

In this group, the hypothalamus calls most of the shots. Then the pituitary, adrenal, and thyroid glands work in complex response to the hypothalamus and to each other. The first step in thyroid activity, then, is receiving a signal through the chain of command. The hypothalamus gives a green light to the pituitary gland, and the pituitary gland creates the first important hormone for thyroid function: thyroid stimulating hormone, or TSH. TSH then goes on to the thyroid gland and lets it know that it's time to do its job.

Having received the TSH signal, the thyroid gland produces T4. T4 floats around in the bloodstream and doesn't do much on its own. What the body really needs to produce energy in its cells is T3. To create T3, the liver pulls on some of the T4 reserve and converts it to T3. As cells use T3, the body detects a decrease in circulating T3 and draws even more from the pool of T4. The hypothalamus notices that T3 and T4 supplies are dwindling, and it starts the process all over again. Problems can arise at any point in this intricate production line, from the very first signal to produce TSH to the conversion of T4 to T3 at the end.

Hypothalamic-Pituitary-Thyroid Axis

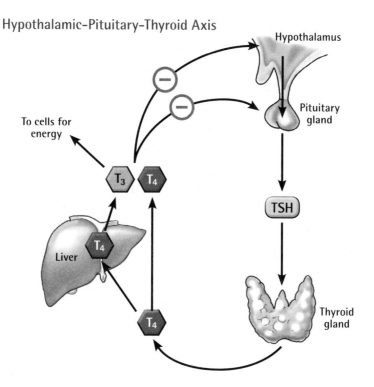

How thyroid function slows down: Hashimoto's thyroiditis, stress, hormones, and more

The first and most prominent way in which thyroid function can be hindered is by the development of Hashimoto's thyroiditis, an autoimmune condition that accounts for the vast majority of hypothyroidism cases. In Hashimoto's, the immune system attacks the thyroid gland, which becomes too damaged to produce sufficient amounts of T4 and T3. This often results in elevated TSH levels, as the hypothalamus and pituitary gland use TSH to beg the unresponsive thyroid gland to produce more hormones.

The body can also develop a problem converting T4 to T3 as a result of stress—both psychological and physiological. Sources of stress that impact thyroid function are emotional stress, restricted food intake, excessive exercise (especially if calories are not sufficiently replenished), restricted carbohydrate intake (typically below 50 to 100 grams per day, though this varies by individual), fasting, and cycles of overeating and undereating. Worse than a simple decline in T3, however, is that stress causes the production of *reverse T3,* a molecule that actively interferes with T3 doing its job. So if you are stressed, your T3 goes down, and whatever T3 you do manage to produce is blocked by reverse T3. It's no wonder that women feel sleepy these days.

You can also have an overabundance of estrogen in your body—a condition called estrogen dominance (see page 270). Excess estrogen interferes with thyroid activity.

Being overweight and/or insulin resistant poses problems for the thyroid gland in a number of different ways. It weighs down bodily systems, increases estrogen levels, induces hyper-insulinemia and inflammation, burdens the liver, and, because of all these components of metabolic brokenness, decreases the body's ability to synthesize T3.

Finally, iodine and/or selenium deficiency can cause thyroid problems. Without iodine, the backbone of T4 and T3 molecules, the thyroid gland can't produce the T4 and T3 you need. Ordinarily, this is not a problem. Most salt in the Western diet is iodized, and both iodine and selenium are abundant in seafood. However, some people consume iodine-free sea salt or iodine-free table salt. Make sure to get enough of both iodine and selenium in your diet by consuming seafood, seaweed, and at least some iodized salt.

Hyperthyroidism

While most women with thyroid problems experience a decrease in thyroid activity, it is possible to suffer from increased thyroid activity. This is called *hyperthyroidism,* and it usually occurs as a result of Graves' disease, an autoimmune condition. In Graves', TSH levels run dangerously low, while T4 and T3 levels are elevated. Symptoms include increased heart rate, weight loss, insatiable appetite, insomnia, and manic energy.

> ## Thyroid health and modern medicine
>
> Piled on top of all these potential thyroid woes is the real kicker: many medical professionals fail to recognize how complex thyroid dysfunction is. When a woman gets her thyroid hormone tested, the doctor normally tests for T4 alone, or for TSH and T4. If T4 is normal, the woman is given a free pass. But what about T3, or even reverse T3? Or Hashimoto's thyroiditis antibodies? T3 is particularly important to check since it is the final test of healthy thyroid function. If you don't know how much of your thyroid hormone in the form of T3 is making it into your cells, then how do you know whether your thyroid system is working as it should?

What to do for hypothyroidism:

○ Get tested for hypothyroidism, including all the hormones: TSH, T4, and T3.

○ Include a test for Hashimoto's thyroiditis antibodies, which will almost always tell you if Hashimoto's is the cause of your hypothyroidism.

If you have Hashimoto's thyroiditis:

○ Eat a gut health and autoimmune disease–friendly diet such as the *Sexy by Nature* diet that emphasizes nourishment and avoids gut irritants such as grains, legumes, and dairy.

○ Include fermented foods or probiotics in your diet to speed gut healing.

○ Experiment with eliminating egg whites, nuts, and the nightshades tomatoes, peppers, potatoes, and eggplant from your diet as well. These foods have been known to aggravate autoimmunity in sensitive individuals.

○ Do not supplement with iodine, which can aggravate the situation. If you are iodine deficient and need to supplement with iodine, however, and under the advisement of a medical professional, be sure to pair it with selenium, which blunts potential aggravation.

○ Reduce stress.

If you do not have Hashimoto's thyroiditis:

○ Reduce stress, which is one of the predominant causes of poor conversion to T3.

○ Consume seafood, which contains both iodine and selenium in replenishing amounts.

○ Consume iodized salt.

○ Consider supplementing with iodine in the form of seaweed consumption or kelp tablets. Consult a physician before doing so.

○ Assure sufficient selenium intake by taking a supplement or eating two Brazil nuts each day.

○ If your blood tests show that you have high estrogen levels or you suspect that you have estrogen dominance, take the steps listed on page 271 to minimize it.

○ Make sure to eat sufficient carbohydrate—at least 100 grams a day, or several servings of vegetables or three pieces of fruit. Your liver needs glucose to convert T4 to T3. If you are an athlete, bump it up to at least 150 grams a day.

○ Increase sleep duration and quality.

○ Stand, walk, sprint, and strength train.

○ Do not over-exercise.

How it works:
blood sugar metabolism and regulation

You can also become fatigued because of poor blood sugar metabolism. As was covered in Step 2, spiking blood sugar by eating meals composed of junky carbohydrates and refined sugar can send your blood sugar plummeting once the sugar high fades. This leads to crankiness, hunger, and fatigue.

Ever feed a child a bag of Skittles and watch her bounce off the walls for forty-five minutes, then zonk out for the following hour? Or experience a seemingly insurmountable urge to sleep after a large meal? Both experiences are the result of a blood sugar high followed by a blood sugar low.

If blood sugar levels do not spike, however, they never plummet, and they never leave you feeling cranky and exhausted.

Blood Sugar After a Meal

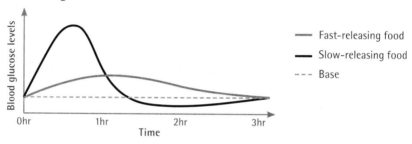

What to do to stabilize blood sugar:

○ Focus on healthful carbohydrates: vegetables, fruits, and the starches listed in Step 2. These foods spike blood sugar and insulin levels less than their processed counterparts, resulting in a gentle blood sugar slope rather than a spike followed by a crash.

○ Pair carbohydrates with fat and protein to reduce sugar spikes.

○ For carbohydrate sources in your diet, focus on vegetables and fruits that are high in fiber and low in glucose, such as leafy greens and berries, rather than starches and rice, which are higher in glucose and have a stronger propensity for spiking blood sugar.

○ If you still react to natural carbohydrates with blood sugar highs and lows, consider minimizing the quantities in which you eat them and dispersing them throughout the day. Eating a little bit of carbohydrate with each meal is better for blood sugar regulation than eating all your carbohydrates at once.

General recommendations for greater energy

○ Reduce stress.

○ Troubleshoot your circadian rhythm with a regular sleep schedule and by manipulating blue and orange light exposure.

○ Stick to natural lighting as much as possible, and expose yourself to blue light during the day.

○ Do your best to wake naturally rather than with an alarm.

○ Troubleshoot thyroid health.

○ Experiment with carbohydrate intake to learn how your blood sugar works.

○ Eat a diet rich in fat and protein to prevent blood sugar spikes.

○ Minimize blood sugar spikes by pairing natural carbohydrates with protein and fat rather than eating sugar-rich snacks.

○ Eat a diet rich in animal products for B vitamin sufficiency, which supports adrenal health and promotes youthful energy.

○ Eat liver and other organ meats for B vitamins, iron, copper, zinc, and other nutrients necessary for energy.

○ Eat seafood for sufficient iodine and selenium.

○ Consider supplementing with a vitamin B complex in the morning (though natural sources such as animal products and especially liver are best).

○ Consider supplementing with cod liver oil, which contains vitamins A and D.

○ Get plenty of sun exposure for vitamin D.

○ Consider supplementing with a 2:1 calcium to magnesium pill for adrenal support.

○ Stop drinking coffee, which impairs your natural ability to have energy.

○ Use healthful carbohydrates such as honey in your tea as an occasional energy booster rather than coffee.

○ Integrate healthy exercise into your life.

○ Stand or walk around most of the day rather than sitting.

Weight Management:
Be slim

The secret to being slim is *quality*. I have said it before, but it bears repeating. Almost nothing in this book bears repeating more. The problem with contemporary weight-loss efforts is that we almost always try to lose weight by reducing the quantity of food we eat. We restrict. We weigh. We measure.

But if you have a broken metabolism, it doesn't matter how much you restrict yourself. It doesn't matter how much you cut back. If you eat garbage, your metabolism will have nothing to work with but garbage. If you eat excellence, however, your metabolism will work excellently.

So that's weight loss in a nutshell. Throw quantity out the window. Throw out diets. Throw out forcing yourself to exercise. Give your body the fuel it needs to fix itself, and watch the pounds melt off. Focusing on quality rather than quantity is the fastest, most efficient, and most permanent way to lose weight. Do calories matter? Somewhat. Are there complexities? Absolutely, especially in a female body. Is there a chance that your weight loss will be slow, or that your weight will plateau at a level higher than you'd like? Yes. But if you give your body what it needs, it will heal itself. In the majority of cases, weight loss is a natural and relatively effortless part of that process. Your body doesn't want to be overweight; it wants to be a healthy weight. It wants to run smoothly. It wants to be radiant. You just have to give it the love and nourishment it deserves.

> Focusing on quality rather than quantity is the fastest, most efficient, and most permanent way to lose weight.

How it works: weight gain

Weight gain is a multifaceted problem. There are perhaps a billion theories on how people gain weight. Some are better than others, obviously. Yet when it comes down to it, they probably all have at least a kernel of truth to them.

The two most popular theories out there today are exactly that way. These two theories don't tell the whole story, but they *almost* get it. A good way to talk about the facts of weight gain and weight loss, therefore, is to take a good, hard look at these theories and explain both how they are correct and how they need tweaking.

The first popular theory is genetics. It says, "Your genes make you fat." This theory is right about the importance of genes, but the way you treat your genes is even more important. Genes are triggered only if the right stimulus is applied. You will gain weight only if you eat the kinds of foods that your genes do not like. For example, if you have a gene that promotes fat storage and you eat French fries, you will gain weight. Eating inflammatory foods such as French fries promotes metabolic brokenness—so you have pulled the genetic trigger. Yet if you have this fat-storing gene and you *don't* eat metabolically damaging foods, but instead choose healthy foods that do not break your metabolism, you will stay lean. Your fat genes will go untriggered. You don't have to become overweight; your genes only make it *possible*. And you don't have to stay overweight; your genes are amenable to change. You are not doomed. You have will. You have agency. You have the ability to work *with* your genes to transform yourself into the healthiest and sexiest woman you can be.

The second popular theory is that calories make you fat. This is also true to an extent. There is a clear correlation between the rise in calorie intake and the expansion of American waistlines over the last several decades. Plus, the whole idea makes intuitive sense: if you eat more energy than your body needs in order to function, then you will have to store it somewhere. It doesn't matter if those extra calories are in the form of carbohydrates, fat, or protein. Excess energy becomes fat, plain and simple. The problem with this theory is that it puts the blame on your shoulders. It's not your fault if your hunger-regulating mechanisms have gone off the rails. When your body no longer sends the right hunger signals, you will naturally overeat, and you will gain weight.

Today, most scientists and doctors advise eating a low-calorie diet. They do so because they believe that limiting calories will prevent you from becoming overweight, which in turn will reduce your risk for disease. In this mindset, calories come first, fat storage comes second, and disease comes third. It's no wonder calories are so important to these people—they think that calories are the primary cause of disease.

The real model for health, however, is more complicated. The real model goes like this: eating low-quality foods leads to overeating and metabolic brokenness, which makes you overweight and sick.

> Eating low-quality foods leads to overeating and metabolic brokenness, which makes you overweight and sick.

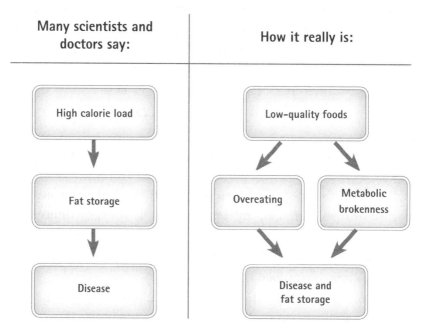

Many scientists and doctors say:

High calorie load

Fat storage

Disease

How it really is:

Low-quality foods

Overeating

Metabolic brokenness

Disease and fat storage

Low-quality foods make you eat too much

Certain foods have greater satiating power than others. This is an easy idea to grasp if you think about a couple of meals. How do you feel after eating a bowl of Ramen noodles, for example, versus a quarter pound of steak and some vegetables? They have the same calorie content, but one meal is empty of nutrition, and the other delivers all the goods. One leaves you wanting more, and the other leaves you satisfied and full. Imagine the difference in your hunger signaling when you eat not just one meal like this, but a lifetime of meals.

Processed foods are the least satisfying of all. In fact, they are deliberately manufactured to leave you hungry, *maybe hungrier than you were before you ate them*. This is how pretzels and chips work (which isn't to say that "healthy" options such as breakfast cereals do not do the same thing). Chips are so good that they are legendary for the simple claim that no one can eat just one. But they don't fill you up. You can eat a whole bag before you know it. Potato chip designers know this, too. They want you to be addicted. They want you to consume as much of their product as possible. So they design it to be as addictive as possible and to override your natural hunger and satiation signals.

Metabolic brokenness

Metabolic brokenness is what happens when all the things that can go wrong in Step 2 of this book do go wrong. If gut flora die, if the gut lining becomes compromised, if the body becomes inflamed, if insulin and leptin signaling are derailed by unhealthy foods, if reproductive hormones run off-track, and if thyroid levels plummet, then your body is going to develop less and less of an ability to metabolize food healthfully.

It almost doesn't matter how many calories you eat at this point. Unnatural foods pollute your body and make it impossible for you to efficiently burn and store fat, metabolize food, obtain nutrients, heal yourself, and maintain a naturally curvy, sexy, and fit figure.

How it works: fat loss

Burning fat takes two things: 1) understanding what can prevent fat-burning in the body and 2) fixing those problems. Fortunately, we have already done the first part—we know what the problems are. The second part is also entirely within your reach. Burning fat requires healing this metabolic brokenness. You heal metabolic brokenness simply by eliminating modern toxins and embracing natural foods. Of course, there are complexities involved, and each woman has her own unique health journey— but the gist of healing is very simple: give your body the nutrients it needs. These nutrients are covered extensively in Step 2. With these natural powerhouses as fuel, your body will heal itself, reduce cravings, and slim down on its own.

If you are still concerned with calories, I can nearly guarantee that switching from a processed diet to a natural one will reduce your calorie intake. Processed foods are insidiously hyper-caloric. Natural foods are not. Natural foods have the right amount of energy and nutrition that you need for a naturally slim and healthy waistline. Can you limit calories or practice moderate fasting in order to speed your weight loss? Quite possibly. Just be careful, and watch what effects your efforts have on both your psychological and physiological wellness. In the long run, it is better to err on the side of healing and natural weight loss than to risk the poor health outcomes associated with drastic dieting.

There's one more crucial factor in fat loss that I haven't touched on yet: the female-specific component. Does estrogen play a role in weight loss? How much fat loss is healthy for women? Is weight loss really more difficult for women than it is for men? Weight loss for women is still all about healing metabolic brokenness—it's just a bit more complicated. Being designed to conceive, carry, and birth babies, women have different amounts and kinds of fat than men do, and we need to take care of our bodies so they do not go into starvation panic and stall our weight-loss efforts. The most effective way to lose weight is to learn about your body's female-specific needs and use them to your advantage.

Female-specific fat needs

As women, we have four special considerations:

1. **Fat is *necessary* for our health and the health of our babies.**

Never forget that fat is necessary for women's health. While a man can go as low as 4 percent body fat without experiencing negative health consequences, a woman should never go below 15 percent. Doing so can result in infertility, low libido, insomnia, depression, anxiety, osteoporosis, and so much more. The female body is designed to store more fat than the male. This assures that babies can be carried to term and have all the energy they need.

Body Fat Ranges for Standard Adults[1,2]

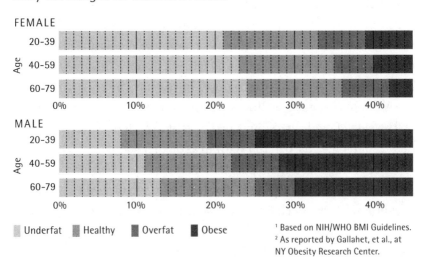

2. **Women have unique fat storage locations that have different health implications.**

   Female fat exists in a number of places. First, it sits beneath the skin all over the body, which explains why women have less muscle definition than men. It also sits in the breasts, buttocks, hips, and thighs. These are healthy fat deposits that you should cherish. The only fat that women really need to be concerned about in terms of health is abdominal fat. Fat around the abdomen in both men and women is the only fat that has been consistently tied to inflammation, insulin resistance, diabetes, and heart disease. Fat on the buttocks, hips, and thighs has not. In fact, female fat significantly boosts fertility, stores nutrients, and makes babies healthier and smarter.

   It is also quite possible to be naturally thin and without much curvature. That's healthy, too. What is important is that you do not deprive yourself of whatever amount of fat your body needs in order to be healthy and strong.

3. **Estrogen influences fat deposition and burning.**

   Female hormones, and especially estrogen, are crucial for maintaining a healthy weight. In excess, however, they can cause weight gain and make it difficult to lose weight. A few particular populations of women are uniquely at risk for estrogen-related fat-burning complications: women who suffer from estrogen dominance, women on birth control pills, and menopausal women.

   Women with inordinately high levels of estrogen in their systems often have a hard time losing weight, as estrogen can promote fat storage. However, estrogen levels usually rise so high as a result of inflammatory diets, stress, and being overweight, so eating the *Sexy by Nature* diet should help mitigate the dominance problem. This is a part of the natural healing with high-quality foods that I have been espousing all along. More specific steps to mitigate estrogen dominance can be found on page 271.

   Women who use hormonal birth control methods may also struggle with weight gain, especially if they take an estrogen-containing formulation of the pill. Weight gain is in fact one of the most common side effects of birth control pills. The only answer to this quandary is to try a different pill formulation—I recommend one with no or little estrogen in this case—or to consider non-hormonal birth control options.

The final population that struggles with weight gain and hormones is menopausal women. The problem for them is not so much estrogen excess as it is estrogen depletion. Estrogen levels fall during menopause. On the surface, decreased estrogen levels might seem like a good thing, since we have seen how estrogen often promotes weight gain. However, having at least some estrogen is crucial for efficient fat-burning. When estrogen levels drop during menopause, it becomes more difficult for many women to stay slim. Moreover, many women experience a shift in *the location* of body fat once they begin menopause. Estrogen directs fat storage toward the hips, buttocks, breasts, and thighs, so lower estrogen levels often result in fat being stored elsewhere, such as in the abdomen. The best you can do in this case is to eat a natural diet (which reduces inflammation and provides the nutritional building blocks you need to synthesize hormones), live with as little stress as possible (since stress reduces pituitary activity), and engage in as much healthy sexual activity as possible (since sexual activity can increase sex hormone production). Additional steps to overcome menopause symptoms can be found on page 243.

4. **Women's bodies cannot tolerate starvation in the same way men's bodies can, and therefore require a focus on nourishment like the *Sexy by Nature* paradigm in order to shed weight efficiently.**

Along with female fat comes a host of mechanisms designed to fight for it. The female body holds onto fat in a way that the male body doesn't. This doesn't mean that weight loss is impossible. To the contrary. Weight loss is eminently possible, but you can't expect it to be as simple or easy as it is for a man, and you have to work *with* your natural fat needs rather than against them.

As a woman, starving yourself can induce weight loss, but it often backfires. The more you restrict yourself, the more your body fights to hang onto fat stores and store even more fat, both at that instant and in the long run. Women who have been on yo-yo diets throughout their lives can probably write whole books on their experiences of this phenomenon. "Success" with conventional diets is fleeting. In the end, weight loss often ends up as weight *gain*. In fact, the body creates new fat cells during periods of starvation. It also actively decreases thyroid activity, which is crucial for energy metabolism and fat-burning. For these reasons, the female body reacts more effectively to healing than it does to dieting. Working *with* the body is the most efficient way to get fat off and keep it off for good.

What to do for weight loss: heal metabolic brokenness and work with the female body

○ **Eat natural foods.** Removing toxins from your diet helps your body heal itself. It almost goes without saying at this point. As your body relaxes into a diet that rejuvenates rather than poisons, it heals.

○ **Reduce stress.** Stress has the ability to inflame your intestinal and hormone environments. It may not have as obvious and immediate an effect as food does, but its impact is every bit as real. Do everything you can to investigate your priorities, organize your life in a more relaxing manner, and take care of yourself.

○ **Sleep more.** Sleep has been shown to dramatically improve insulin and leptin signaling. Without adequate sleep, otherwise healthy people fairly quickly develop the same hormone profiles as pre-diabetics. Cravings also increase in a state of sleep deprivation. For these reasons, many researchers have hypothesized that poor sleep is one of the primary causes of American illness and obesity.

Sleep as much as you can, and do your best to wake naturally after a full night's sleep. If that's not possible, or if you end up getting less sleep than you should one night, follow that night with a lower-carbohydrate breakfast, since you have less insulin sensitivity, and with forgiveness for your body as it craves more food and especially sweet foods throughout the next sleepy day.

o **Heal your gut and support healthy gut bacteria.** Aside from simply eating natural foods, it may be helpful to focus on healing your gut, since poor gut flora health can contribute to insulin resistance. Do this first by steering clear of inflammatory foods such as grains, legumes, and dairy, and second by consuming either fermented foods or a probiotic supplement daily.

o **Consider a lower-carbohydrate diet.** Diets low in carbohydrate often radically improve insulin sensitivity and weight loss in overweight women. Perhaps a low-carbohydrate diet is right for you. Start with a diet that relies on vegetables as its primary carbohydrate source. Without dense carbohydrates like fruit or starches in your diet, insulin levels will inevitably fall, and the fat-burning capacity of glucagon can kick in more effectively. Note that athletes need to eat more carbohydrates than less-active women do—a *minimum* of 50 to 100 grams of dense carbohydrate each day.

o **If that doesn't work for you, consider a lower-fat diet.** Low-fat diets have also been shown to promote weight loss. Don't consciously restrict calories or fat in a way that is psychologically harmful. Yet if it comes easily for you to reduce fat to 50 to 80 grams per day, doing so can reduce your caloric load and help your body burn fat as fuel.

o **Limit dairy.** Dairy is a highly insulinogenic food and can significantly hamper weight-loss and insulin-sensitizing efforts.

o **Eat in meals.** Grazing and snacking are habits that prevent your body from being able to run through all its excess energy stores. Insulin levels remain elevated, and glucagon cannot burn fat.

o **Exercise, specifically by sprinting and strength training.** Exercise can be a great tool for weight loss. Not only does it promote muscle growth, fat-burning during a workout, and fat-burning afterward, but it also makes you feel healthier, happier, and more energized.

Focus on sprint-based exercises, which have the unique ability to sharpen insulin sensitivity. Weight-training is also great for fat-burning since it promotes muscle growth, and muscle tissue demands a lot of calories even at rest. Steer clear of chronic, monotonous cardio exercise, which does little to improve metabolic fitness.

○ **Consider consuming or supplementing with natural fat-burning boosters.** Many vitamins, minerals, and foods promote metabolic fitness and fat-burning. Magnesium, zinc, and chromium all may promote insulin sensitivity. Vitamin C and all the B vitamins, especially vitamin B_{12}, also promote healthy insulin signaling and weight management. These nutrients are abundant in the *Sexy by Nature* diet, but supplementing with them can give you a powerful boost, especially in the case of magnesium, which is particularly hard to come by in the modern diet.

Coconut is a fat-burning superfood. Coconut is composed primarily of medium-chain fatty acids, which are complicated, but about which you need to know only that they are burned incredibly efficiently by mitochondria, the "engines" of cells. When it replaces other oils in the diet, coconut oil has been shown to improve metabolic fitness and fat loss.

○ **Eat when you are hungry, and stop when you are full.** Can it really be that easy? Yes. Eat natural foods when you are hungry and stop when you are full, and your metabolism will right itself on its own. It may take some time—I understand that navigating hunger and knowing when it's appropriate to eat is difficult for a lot of women—but this truly is one of the most helpful means to promote weight loss.

○ **Accept and account for your female hormones.** I am not a nature idealist—I do not advocate *Sexy by Nature* just because I love natural bodies. I advocate living and eating this way because it is the only way that really *works*. *Sexy by Nature* is not just the healthiest but also the most efficient and long-lasting way to lose weight.

Female hormones are tricky, and they are very powerful. For that reason, we have to work *with* rather than against them. The right way to do so is somewhat slowly. Have patience. If your progress seems too slow at times, remember that the alternative is far worse. No one wants to be infertile, sexless, and covered in acne. I've been there.

As you lose weight, you might hit a plateau, especially if you are obese. An overweight woman will in all likelihood melt down to a healthy, sexy weight within the normal range of body fat percentages. If you are obese, however, or if you have other health struggles on your plate along with weight to lose, you may find that your weight loss stalls at a higher plateau or takes longer than you'd like. Still, if you achieve healthy blood markers and a healthy metabolism and happen to be a few body fat percentage points overweight rather than several dozen, then you are *healthy,* and you should stop comparing yourself to body fat charts that cannot account for your unique body and situation.

As you continue your weight-loss journey, the most important thing to do is to take context into account. You have a unique shape, size, and story. You have fat in different places than other women, and different amounts of it. You have different hormone levels. You will have a different path. The trick is to accept where you are, set reasonable goals, and love and forgive yourself as you move forward, while feeling excited about the greater health and sexiness you are achieving.

In our culture, we can't help but associate a slimmer waistline with being sexy. But far more than that, being sexy is about health. It is about being *fertile.* It's about life and vitality and loving your body. It's about having a sex drive. Having energy. Having curves. Having clear skin and bright eyes. Being feminine and radiant and happy. These things are not secondary to body fatness. They are other indicators of health that should not be forgotten in the quest for weight loss, and they are equally crucial for turning your body into a healthy home in which you are happy to live.

Skin Health:
Be radiant

Contrary to the popular dermatology mantra that lotions solve everything and food solves nothing, there is nothing more powerful for skin health than improving the quality of your diet. If you eat garbage, your cells will swim in it, and they are not going to be able to help it if they get red and sick. If you eat nutrient-dense foods and support healthy hormone function with an anti-inflammatory diet, your skin will heal, glow, and radiate.

How it works: skin

The skin is the largest organ in the body. It is also one of the key players in keeping you toxin-free, as it is the primary barrier between you and the outside world. If you have skin disturbances, it is completely understandable, and you are definitely not alone. The skin does a lot of heavy lifting, and in this toxic, inflamed world, it's no wonder that this incredibly multifaceted and important organ often struggles to keep up.

The skin is composed of three layers: the epidermis, which is the thinnest of the three layers and sits on the very top; the dermis, which sits in the middle; and the hypodermis, which connects skin to bone and muscle. Contrary to logic, the epidermis—the layer everyone gets to see—is not all that important. It is composed of dead skin cells that are in a constant state of being sloughed off and replenished. This process takes approximately 35 days.

The real action takes place in the middle layer, the dermis. This is where collagen provides firmness to the skin and where hair follicles, sweat glands, nerve endings, and blood vessels reside. Most important for acne sufferers, inside the dermis sit the sebaceous glands, which secrete oil onto the surface of the skin. This oil normally performs a good, protective function. In excess, however, it can create oily skin and acne. When inflamed, it exacerbates acne and leads to skin disorders such as eczema and rosacea.

Topical elements can affect your skin, too. You can abrade your skin with harsh chemicals, for example. But far and away the most important thing you can do is to correct the problems of hormone imbalance and inflammation from the inside out.

Acne in three steps: hormones, inflammation, and infection

Conventional dermatological wisdom is that bacteria are the primary cause of acne. This has a grain of truth to it, since bacteria do play a role, but it is minimal compared to the internal conditions that start acne in the first place. Acne in reality develops in three steps. First, male sex hormones can cause excess oil production in the dermis layer of the skin, which clogs pores (though surface debris can also clog pores, rendering hormones less important). Second, inflammation attacks the clogged pores. Third, bacteria infect the clogged pores and cause low-level inflammation to increase to large, painful, irritated pustules. The two primary causes of acne are hormone balance and inflammation; bacteria are only a tertiary concern.

Male sex hormones can dominate female sex hormones in the blood a number of ways. Insulin resistance, blood sugar spikes, stress, starvation diets, and the menstrual cycle are all potential culprits, many of which often occur simultaneously. It is also possible for progesterone (a female sex hormone) to cause acne; this occurs as a result of the menstrual cycle and birth control pills.

Insulin resistance and hormone imbalance

Insulin resistance gives millions of women hormonal acne. It occurs via a simple mechanism: insulin stimulates testosterone production in the ovaries. Chronically elevated insulin levels lead to chronically elevated testosterone. Testosterone is a male sex hormone that directly stimulates oil production in pores. If you are insulin resistant and experience acne, testosterone is likely a primary contributor to your acne woes. This explains why so many women with polycystic ovarian syndrome experience acne. High testosterone is one of the primary characteristics of PCOS.

Blood sugar and hormone imbalance

Blood sugar spikes contribute to acne largely because they elicit an insulin response, which in turn spikes testosterone production (in addition to causing inflammation). This phenomenon is not confined to women—it occurs in men as well. It is so common, in fact, that it partly explains why many people break out around the holidays—large quantities of sugary foods lead to blood sugar disasters. It is also part of the reason why many people have skin reactions to dairy, particularly milk: dairy is highly insulinogenic.

Stress and hormone imbalance

Stress is a major player in skin health, and for a wide variety of reasons.

First, the skin contains stress-hormone receptors. When you are stressed out, your skin knows it. It has the ability to panic under stress just as much as your brain does.

Stress is also inflammatory. It inflames the gut, incites the immune system, and makes the skin leap into overdrive. This point is brief, but it is a big deal and needs to be taken seriously. Both psychological and physiological stress contributes to inflammation in a big way.

Finally, stress performs a function in the body known as *pregnenolone steal*. In this process, the stress glands steal the hormonal resource pregnenolone that would otherwise be devoted to making estrogen and other female hormones and instead directs its use to stress hormones such as DHEA-S. This is problematic not only because estrogen has a balancing effect against testosterone and is great for your skin, but also because DHEA-S acts similarly to testosterone with respect to the skin and stimulates oil production.

Starvation and hormone imbalance

The reproductive system does not like being toyed with, so denying it nourishment does not go over well. Restricting calories, exercising too much, and radically depleting fat stores are three surefire ways to signal starvation.

The female sex hormones estrogen and progesterone are hit particularly hard by these starvation signals, which is unfortunate, because estrogen is one of the most powerful molecules for healthy skin. If estrogen levels decrease far enough relative to testosterone or DHEA-S, acne often results. It is also worth noting that estrogen is produced in fat cells. If your fat stores fall below a healthy level, your estrogen levels may end being up too low for healthy skin.

The menstrual cycle and hormone imbalance

Many women experience breakouts in connection with their monthly cycles. Unfortunately, hormone balance functions differently in different women, so I can't make any overarching statements about the precise events occurring in your body. However, there are some clues I can point to.

The first two weeks of the menstrual cycle, which include the week of bleeding and the following week, are generally quite calm for women and entail great skin health. At the two-week mark, however, or during ovulation, testosterone levels spike. For women for whom oil production is a problem, or for whom testosterone levels are already out of balance from insulin resistance and the like, ovulation can cause acne outbreaks.

The second half of the menstrual cycle can be problematic, too. Estrogen and progesterone levels fall and rise in delicate balance throughout this time. If one leaps out ahead of the other or drops through the basement, skin changes can occur. Estrogen is generally regarded as a balm for the skin. In contrast, unnaturally elevated progesterone causes acne. What is the best thing you can do to reduce monthly breakouts? Achieve better balance between testosterone, estrogen, and progesterone by eating an anti-inflammatory, hormone-balancing diet like the *Sexy by Nature* diet.

Birth control pills and hormone imbalance

Because all these hormone irregularities can lead to acne, many women begin taking hormonal birth control in the hope of clearing their skin. Sometimes it works. But sometimes it doesn't, and instead makes it much worse. For this reason, some women go through several different pills before finding one with the "right" combination of estrogen and progesterone that enables them to have clear skin. Others never achieve clear skin on birth control, but accept acne as a necessary component of their birth control regimen. This is unnecessary. Not only do several dozen birth control options exist, but a few of them require no hormonal interference at all. The vast diversity of birth control options is explored in depth beginning on page 257.

Inflammation

Acne is perhaps the most visible symptom of systemic inflammation. If you have significant acne, you inevitably have some amount of inflammation in your blood. Without inflammation, the pores clogged by hormones would never become the nasty lumps they are, or at least they would not be quite so big.

For this reason, healing your gut and reducing inflammation are perhaps the most powerful steps you can take to overcome acne. Focusing on inflammation-fighting antioxidants both in your diet (such as those found in fruits and vegetables) and in your skincare routine will go a long way toward soothing your acne. Both supplemental and topical antioxidant use has been shown to reduce breakouts by as much as 50 percent.

Bacteria's role in acne: not guilty!

Bacteria live in and around the layers of everybody's skin. Many dermatologists insist that the key to clear skin is killing off these bacteria, so most topical acne treatments do just that. The thing is, not only do bacteria exist naturally all over the surface of everybody's skin, but they can actively promote skin health.

Sure, it is true that bacteria infect clogged pores. But this is only the case if the bacteria on your skin are in an unhealthy state. The role bacteria play in acne is much like the role they play in the gut: there are both "good" and "bad" bacteria on your skin. You can develop acne only if you have a significant imbalance between good and bad, which occurs as a result of both topical and internal stressors.

Many strains of harmful bacteria are present almost exclusively on the skin of people who have acne relative to those who don't, which demonstrates that bad bacteria are the ones responsible for infecting pores. Even more remarkably, some healthy strains of bacteria are present only on the skin of people who do *not* have acne. This indicates that good bacteria can actually fight acne. Topical probiotics may soon become an important component of skincare regimens, and some are already on the market.

Other skin conditions

Like acne, eczema and rosacea are common torments. They are multifaceted problems that have many causes, likely centered around inflammation and a hyperactive immune response, allergies, and nutrient deficiencies (such as vitamin A). To this end, a diet that emphasizes gut-healing foods, reduces inflammation, and supports immune health is one of the best offenses against both of these often-debilitating problems.

External influences: the role of touching, picking, cleansers, and lotions

Counterintuitive as it might sound, one of the best things you can do for your skin is to stop washing it.

Much like with food, today's culture has this idea that skincare products designed in a laboratory are better for us than natural methods. The chemical barrage to which we subject our skin on a daily basis is unnecessary and often harmful. First, consider the fact that benzoyl peroxide, one of the most popular topical acne treatments available over the counter, reduces antioxidant activity in the skin. Antioxidants are crucial for reducing inflammation. Consider too that the skin has natural oils and cleaning and healing processes that work delightfully well on their own. Washing the skin removes those natural oils, so the skin often dries out in response. When skin is dry, women often turn to lotion. However, the skin also tries to rectify the dryness on its own by increasing oil production. At this point, both you and your skin are engaged in efforts to increase lubrication. Too much lubrication clogs pores, so your washing and moisturizing routine is counterproductive.

The act of washing your face can make it either too dry or too oily, depending on how your skin reacts. Rarely does washing leave skin in tip-top shape. And moisturizers that contain unnatural chemicals often don't heal the skin; they just cover it up. Many natural alternatives to washing and moisturizing, such as apple cider vinegar, baking soda, coconut oil, lard, cod liver oil, and vitamin blends provide real healing to the skin and can be protective in times of dryness or oiliness.

In all fairness, there are probably some manufactured toiletries that do not aggravate your skin. It is not absolutely necessary to "go all natural" and expressly forbid cosmetics. It is only important to note that they can be problematic and to do your best to find products—natural or not—that work for you.

In my experience, the only way to know whether a lotion, if you choose to use one, is a good match for your skin is to try it for a few days and see. A different, more specific test is to apply lotion to one side of your face and not the other in order to witness its effects, or to apply it to the sensitive skin on your wrist or neck before using it on your face. I do not forbid using any manufactured cosmetic products—in fact, I use a lotion that I buy at a mall. But it took me a long time to find one that did not irritate my skin. I opted to use it because it has white tea extract in it, and white tea is a powerful antioxidant. Applying antioxidants such as white tea, green tea, vitamin C, and B vitamins can help reduce inflammation as long as you are certain that you have found a lotion that does not aggravate your skin.

Another way to aggravate your skin is to pick at it. Just as with scabs and wounds, the skin does best when it heals on its own. Have you ever noticed that breakouts often occur near each other? This is because wounds act as beacons for inflammatory molecules. The more aggravated a wound is, the stronger the inflammatory response becomes, so pimples become bigger and nastier the more you touch them. Even worse is the fact that picking causes new pimples to crop up around old ones. Keeping your hands off your face is one of the harder habits to practice, but the less you touch your blemishes, the more your skin will thank you.

Even the simple act of touching clear skin can lead to the development of acne. Fingers carry all kinds of bacteria, dirt, and oils. When you touch your face, you put these dirty oils directly in contact with your pores. When I was in high school and college, I always had acne around my mouth, particularly on the right side of my face. It took me years to realize that I was breaking out because I rested my chin on my hand while I studied. Once I broke that habit, the acne faded away.

What to do for radiant skin

○ Eliminate sugar and insulinogenic foods and focus on reducing inflammation.

○ Eliminate gut-irritating foods such as grains, legumes, and dairy.

○ Include gut-healing foods such as fermented foods, or consider probiotic supplements.

○ If you eat a lot of fiber, consider reducing the amount of fiber in your diet, particularly insoluble fiber. Lots of fiber can irritate your gut lining if you are already dealing with inflammation or a sensitive gut.

○ Keep protein intake on the lower end of the spectrum—at 50 to 75 grams per day. Excess protein is a key player in oil production and oxidation.

○ Eliminate (or experiment with) hormonal influences on your skin. The most important hormonal foods are dairy, particularly milk, and phytoestrogens, especially flax and soy.

○ Eat to meet the needs of your metabolism. Estrogen levels are at their best when you assure your body that it is being properly fed.

○ Consume plenty of fat to assure adequate collagen stores.

○ Consume at least three servings of fatty fish such as salmon every week. Alternatively, consider supplementing with cod liver oil, which delivers vitamins A and D—crucial vitamins for healthy skin—as well as anti-inflammatory omega-3 fatty acids.

○ Eat liver on a regular basis. Liver is the densest source of vitamin A available in the human diet.

○ Consume homemade bone broth—that is, broth made from simmering bones in water—which is rich in collagen, calcium, magnesium, and other nutrients necessary for skin health.

○ Consume a diet rich in antioxidants, such as leafy greens and other vegetables and fruits.

•

○ Exercise.

○ Manage your specific health issue. PCOS and hypothyroidism are particularly problematic when it comes to skin health: PCOS because of its hormonal effects, and hypothyroidism simply because cells lack the energy they need to heal.

○ Discontinue the use of soaps and abrasive cleansers, consider natural alternatives to conventional products, or make your own remedies from natural ingredients such as baking soda, coconut oil, and olive oil. Store-bought alternatives may work fine. The trick is to find one that works for you.

○ Consider using a topical probiotic spray on your skin. Topical probiotics add good bacteria to your skin that have the ability to offset the bad bacteria that inflame pores.

○ Consider applying an antioxidant lotion that includes green tea, white tea, vitamin C, or B vitamins.

○ Exfoliate with a clean washcloth once a week.

○ Do not pick at your skin.

○ Sleep on a clean pillowcase.

○ Keep sunburns and harsh sun exposure to a minimum.

○ Consider supplementing with zinc, an antioxidant that has been shown to be particularly helpful for clear skin. N-acetylcysteine, milk thistle extract, and selenium have also been shown to have powerful effects on skin.

○ Consider supplementing or focusing on other nutrients that are crucial for skin health, such as vitamin A, vitamin C, vitamin E, omega-3 fatty acids, sulfur, B vitamins (particularly niacin), and vitamin K.

Menopause and Aging:
Be youthful

The current condition and future prospects of the Baby Boomer generation are sad and foreboding. While Americans now live longer than humans ever have, we are also becoming immobile sooner in life. A higher proportion of senior citizens are bedridden or wheelchair bound than ever before, and *sooner in life than they used to be*. The modern world as such appears to have created a new phase of human life. No longer do people go right from living well to passing on. Squeezed between adulthood and death is a new, decades-long phase of immobility and disease. This discussion doesn't even touch on the Alzheimer's issue, which has skyrocketed to prominence not just because it's more easily diagnosed these days but also because more and more seniors (and older adults) are retaining less and less of their memory.

How it works: aging

The current, erroneous way of thinking about aging is that it's inevitable. Bodies fall apart over time, don't they? Well, they do, a bit. But don't you know of at least a few older athletes? Vibrant centenarian yogis? Elderly neighbors who still walk several miles a day and maintain their own gardens? Aging for them doesn't look like the traditional American model. Instead, it is a continuation of vibrant life and health.

We could argue that these people are lucky, but I don't think that's the case. Death is inevitable, but aging the way we do today is not. Aging with pain, sickness, and disease is not natural—it is the result of damage done to the body over time.

If you continually put your body through the wringer, it will break down faster. For example, insulin resistance doesn't just *happen* one day for no reason. You have a much greater chance of developing insulin resistance as an elderly person than as a child. This is why type 2 diabetes used to be called adult-onset diabetes: it developed slowly over time. Obesity doesn't just happen. Heart disease doesn't just happen. Alzheimer's doesn't just happen. All these conditions build up incrementally.

Being inflamed for a lifetime tires a body out. It falls apart in some way. Of course degeneration occurs naturally over time, but to the degree that it does today? Hardly. It doesn't have to be this way. If we don't stress our bodies, don't inflame them, treat them with love and care, and work with them, then we set up the best possible defense.

What to do for youthfulness

○ **Nourish yourself.** Many health problems are associated with aging. Achy joints, arthritis, varicose veins, glaucoma, diverticulitis, insulin resistance, dementia, and cancer are just a few.

Whole books are written to address these problems—there is no way I can do any of them justice here. The best I can say is that consuming an anti-inflammatory, nutrient-rich diet of natural and organic animal products—including organ meats—that keeps sugar to a minimum and eschews alcohol and smoking is perhaps the best thing you can do.

○ **Fast.** There has been a fair bit of hype in recent years about the benefits of fasting and low-calorie diets for prolonging life. This may be true—periodic or intermittent fasting may enact metabolic processes that keep the body running smoother longer. There are many different fasting methods. For example, you can confine your eating period to ten hours so that you "fast" for the other fourteen hours of the day. Another option is to fast on alternate days, which might mean eating just one meal every other day and eating freely on off days. The final common means by which to achieve this effect is not to undertake a specific fasting regimen but rather to eat a limited number of calories—perhaps around 1,200 every day.

Think of your body as an engine. If the engine doesn't run so hot all the time, it will be able to run a little bit longer. However, undertaking a fasting or calorie-restricted eating pattern at this point in your life can be psychologically challenging and may not be worth it, especially since its life-lengthening effects may be negligible.

○ **Consider a low-carbohydrate diet.** Many natural health advocates believe that a low-carbohydrate diet that keeps insulin levels low mimics the life-expanding effects of low-calorie dieting and fasting without the psychological and potential physiological hardship. However, I strongly recommend that women of reproductive age who wish to remain fertile and have proper hormone balance tread carefully with restrictive eating patterns, which includes both fasting and extremely low-carbohydrate diets. These methods might minimally prolong life, but they do so to the detriment of reproductive fitness. These recommendations may be best suited to women beyond reproductive age.

○ **Get happy.** The final and most important point worth considering in the *Sexy by Nature* perspective on aging is the role of happiness. While diet and lifestyle changes are crucial components of a long and healthy life for most people, peace, happiness, and a sense of purpose may be even more important. Consider all the vibrant elderly people you know. Do they not all have goals, practices, or passions around which they orient their lives, or at least a profound sense of community, peace, and love? Few places in *Sexy by Nature* demonstrate the power of a healthy psychological life more clearly than this one. Happiness is *happiness,* so it's great in itself. But happiness is also one of the primary determinants of physical health and vibrant longevity.

How it works: menopause

Menopause is often the first real aging roadblock that women run into. Unlike many other factors of aging, menopause is inevitable. This is because it helps preserve the species. When women stop having their own children, they become grandmothers. Grandmothers, it turns out, are highly advantageous from an evolutionary perspective. Grandmothers ease the burden of childcare for mothers, help mothers bear greater numbers of children, and assure the safety and health of grandchildren. Grandmothers proved themselves so beneficial to human societies that menopause cemented itself as a part of the female genome. Women are meant to continue to be wise, strong, and productive assets of society. Menopause is nature's way of facilitating that behavior.

So menopause is natural. It is good, and it is liberating in many regards. The difficulty with which women often experience it today is heartbreakingly unnecessary.

Menopause is defined by the cessation of ovarian activity that produces a menstrual cycle. It typically occurs between the ages of 40 and 58, with 51 being the average. All irregularities that occur before this point fall under the umbrella of *perimenopause—* though symptoms of perimenopause and menopause are usually quite similar.

Symptoms associated with menopause and perimenopause include heavy menstrual bleeding, hot flashes, night sweats, pain during intercourse, anxiety, irritability, vaginal dryness, low libido, joint pain, frequent urination, a resurgence of acne, and insomnia. Many menopausal women also experience symptoms of male-dominant hormone imbalance, such as male-pattern hair growth and male-pattern hair loss. A common effect is weight gain, particularly in the abdomen. Many women describe a relocation of fat stores from feminine areas such as breasts, hips, and thighs to the abdomen, largely as a result of declining estrogen levels. Menopause is not for sissies.

Most of these symptoms are due to low estrogen and/or progesterone levels. Losing female hormone function is the hallmark cause and condition of menopause. In order for the menstrual cycle to cease, ovarian estrogen and progesterone production decline throughout menopause. Levels of male sex hormones such as testosterone decline, too, but at variable rates. Menopause is best tolerated when the decline occurs steadily over time and across all hormones as equally as possible. Things go wrong and symptoms become extreme when one hormone plummets relative to the others. This is most often the case when estrogen levels drop, leading to most of the symptoms listed above.

Symptoms of menopause are exacerbated by:

○ stress, which reduces progesterone and estrogen production

○ extreme consumption of soy and flax (plant estrogens), which can either reduce estrogen production or significantly elevate estrogen over progesterone and thereby cause symptoms of estrogen dominance

○ weight gain, which may also cause symptoms of estrogen dominance

○ blood sugar swings and insulin resistance, which increase testosterone levels relative to estrogen and progesterone

○ inflammation, which is antagonistic to the management of the delicate flux of hormones during menopause

What to do for menopause

○ Eliminate processed sugars and consider lowering carbohydrate intake to minimize insulin levels and support healthy weight maintenance.

○ Promote healthy gut flora and insulin sensitivity with an anti-inflammatory diet and fermented foods or probiotics.

○ Reduce stress to increase progesterone and estrogen levels.

o Experiment with phytoestrogen intake. If you consume phytoestrogens (particularly flax and soy), consider eliminating them and monitor the effects. On the other hand, if you eat cleanly without these compounds and suffer menopause symptoms, try consuming them to see if they mitigate your symptoms. Some women find that they do.

o Supplement with magnesium to help the uptake of the remaining estrogen into tissues.

o Insomniacs take note: magnesium supplements can significantly aid menopause-related sleep disturbances. They also support healthy hormone production.

o Exercise to increase serotonin and dopamine levels in the brain, which can support healthy sleep, a robust sex drive, and mental health, and to sharpen insulin sensitivity and support healthy weight maintenance.

o Eat a diet rich in protein, vitamin C, and B vitamins to support neurotransmitter health, which can boost libido and reduce anxiety and depression.

o Engage in as much pleasurable sexual and romantic activity as possible, which can boost female sex hormone production.

o Turn to low-dose bio-identical hormone replacement as a last resort. Tread carefully: hormone-replacement estrogen supplementation has questionable effects on the body. It may be linked to the development of breast cancer and other female cancers as well as heart attack and stroke.

Fertility:
Be fruitful

According to the Centers for Disease Control and Prevention, 10 percent of American women seek medical advice related to infertility during their reproductive years.[25] While many complications can play a role, such as fallopian tube disorders or an abnormal uterus, which together account for one-third of infertility cases, millions of other cases are directly related to diet and lifestyle issues.

Even if you have never been diagnosed with conditions that characterize diet- and lifestyle-induced infertility, the hormone misfiring that causes them can crop up in anyone. For example, you may not have been diagnosed with polycystic ovarian syndrome (PCOS), but you may have evaded a diagnosis simply because you have not yet attempted to conceive. Additionally, if you do not have PCOS but do have issues with insulin resistance, then taking the same steps that a woman with insulin-resistant PCOS does may be the extra push you need to make your fertility function as smoothly and efficiently as a Swiss clock. These steps may also relieve you of any symptoms of PCOS that you might exhibit, such as cystic acne.

As I mentioned, a variety of the physiological problems that can lead to infertility cannot be addressed by diet and lifestyle. These problems require specific medical attention and should be ruled out if you are having trouble conceiving. Outside of these conditions, however, there are many causes of infertility that can be overcome naturally. They are usually classified into specific conditions such as PCOS, hypothalamic amenorrhea, and female athletic triad syndrome. These conditions often overlap—a woman can suffer more than one cause of infertility at a time. To that end, the following paragraphs are categorized by diet and lifestyle factors that lead to infertility issues: insulin resistance (often manifesting as PCOS), stress and the body's starvation response (often manifesting as hypothalamic amenorrhea or female athletic triad syndrome), hypothyroidism, and hormonal birth control.

The role of insulin in infertility

The role of insulin resistance in infertility is simple: the presence of insulin in the bloodstream causes the ovaries to produce testosterone. With chronically elevated insulin levels, as is usually the case in a woman who is insulin resistant, diabetic, overweight, or obese, there is more testosterone coursing through the bloodstream than is healthy. Testosterone interferes with the development of healthy follicles—precursors to eggs—and often causes small cysts to develop all over the ovaries. The formation of these cysts is called polycystic ovarian syndrome. It is estimated that approximately 10 percent of women of reproductive age in America have PCOS, making it the most common hormonal disorder among women in this age group.[26] Despite the ubiquity of PCOS, however, it is still possible to suffer from insulin's effects without having an official diagnosis. Symptoms of insulin-induced infertility include acne, male-pattern hair growth, male-pattern hair loss, oily skin, being overweight, and difficulty losing weight.

When women have high testosterone levels, they sometimes have low estrogen levels as well. This makes the hormone imbalance all the more problematic, since estrogen and testosterone function as counterweights in the female body. Without estrogen, testosterone's negative side effects can go unchecked. Yet even in women with high estrogen levels (which is often the case in overweight women because estrogen is produced by fat cells), high testosterone levels can be disruptive enough to impede the development of healthy follicles and create cysts. The power that chronically elevated insulin levels (not the healthy spikes that occur on a diet of natural foods) has to impede the menstrual cycle and halt ovulation and menstruation cannot be understated.

The role of stress in infertility

Stress is a powerful impediment to fertility. Why? Because the female body is designed to respond to positive environments. The body gives a green light for reproduction only when all the criteria for birthing a healthy baby in a healthy environment are met. If you are under any kind of duress, your body reads it as a sign that it's not the right time to reproduce, and it shuts down reproductive activity.

One powerful example of this in nature is the extreme degree of impaired fertility that researchers have witnessed in non-human primates. In one study, across more than 1,200 menstrual cycles in cynomolgus monkeys, the stressed-out, socially subordinate monkeys consistently experienced irregular cycles and fertility problems, while their more popular peers did not. In primate societies, much as in our own, being at the bottom of the social ladder is inherently stressful. For the socially subordinate monkeys in this study, cycles increased in length and variability, and levels of both progesterone and estrogen dropped. They also experienced elevated cortisol levels. The researchers tested soy on the monkeys to see if the plant estrogen would help, and it did not.

It is important to note that these monkeys were not energetically stressed. They did not exercise. They ate the same amount of food as their more popular peers. The only thing that had the power to change their reproductive capacity was psychological stress, and it made a significant impact.[27] These same problems occur in women.

* * *

Under stress, progesterone levels specifically, but also estrogen levels, decrease by another powerful mechanism called *pregnenolone steal,* which I mentioned briefly in the section on skin health. In times of stress, the body shunts hormonal resources away from unnecessary functions like reproduction and toward functions that are more important for survival, such as the production of the stress hormones adrenaline, cortisol, and DHEA-S.

If you are healthy and under a manageable amount of stress, your body will balance hormone resources between reproduction and stress. If you are chronically stressed, however, then your body will produce more stress hormones and less progesterone. Without sufficient progesterone, the body is unable to menstruate or ovulate and becomes infertile.

Worse is the fact that the adrenal hormone DHEA-S acts as an *androgen,* or male sex hormone, in many bodily functions. So not only does pregnenolone steal cause infertility, but it also gives rise to male-pattern symptoms not unlike those created by insulin resistance. Acne, male-pattern hair growth, and male-pattern hair loss might ensue. Ovaries may even become polycystic due to a significant dose of DHEA-S.

The role of starvation in infertility

Starvation crops up a number of times in this book, and for good reason. When your body thinks that it's starving, it stops reproducing. This response made an enormous amount of sense in ancient history. If food was scarce, it was best to wait to conceive until food was more bountiful. In the event of starvation, the female body does its best to promote health and assure the health of future offspring. By shutting down pituitary function, the starvation response is a powerful defense mechanism and means by which to stunt fertility.

Ways to cause infertility with starvation signals include:

○ Eating less food than you need to maintain a healthy weight over an extended period.

○ Deliberately fasting, going significant periods without eating, waiting too long past hunger signals to eat, insisting on a "really hungry" feeling before eating, yo-yo dieting, cycling through bouts of overeating and undereating, filling the stomach with low-calorie foods like vegetables without eating enough fat, protein, or carbohydrate to satisfy calorie needs, or participating in other restrictive behaviors.

○ Burning more calories through exercise than you consume throughout the day.

○ Exercising too often or at excessive intensities.

○ Having too low a percentage of body fat, such as below 15 percent. (The precise value varies for every woman.)

○ Losing body fat too quickly.

Leptin and your body fat set point

One final way to cause starvation signals in your body is to lose too much body fat relative to what your body is used to. This factor is context specific and varies from woman to woman, though it explains why women at different body fat levels have diverse experiences with infertility.

You may have noticed that some women are perfectly fertile at low body weights whereas others are not. This is partially a result of DNA. It is also a matter of environment and what your hormones are used to.

For example, some women who have been rail thin and starved their entire lives, such as many who live on the African savanna, remain perfectly fertile. Yet many women in developed countries may not be able to go below 18 percent body fat without hindering their fertility. Why? Because the women on the savanna have always been rail thin, and most women in industrialized countries have not.[28] Leptin (the hormone secreted by fat cells) is responsible. In response to the environment, each woman's body develops its own leptin set point.

Your brain needs to hear leptin signals properly and loudly enough—and therefore be leptin sensitive—to be satisfied that you are not living in famine. You will not be fertile unless you meet your body's minimum leptin requirements. Does this mean that overweight women can't lose weight without sacrificing their fertility? No. It means that weight loss cannot be too fast or drastic, and that leptin resistance must be overcome by healthy diet and lifestyle choices.

The starvation signal is all about context. Every woman's body reacts differently to leptin, dieting, exercise, and fasting, and every woman's body has its own hormonal environment. Many women who are overweight can go long periods without eating and achieve beneficial results. Fasting can be an excellent way to lose weight in the short term for some women. But if it goes on for too long or is too extreme, the body may start reading these behaviors as starvation events.

The healthiest thing you can do for your body is to eat when you are hungry and stop eating when you are full. If it takes you a long time to get hungry again after a meal and you feel happy waiting, then continue. It is your body, and it's your job to listen and give it the fuel it needs.

Signs of overdoing it include:

○ Fading or absent menstrual cycles

○ Low libido

○ Vaginal dryness

○ Anxiety

○ Insomnia

○ A fasting "high" or an overabundance of energy when you do not eat

○ Irritability when you are hungry

○ Obsessive thoughts about food

○ Fatigue

○ Constant hunger

Compounding stress: experiencing physical and psychological stress together

Worse than physical or psychological stress in isolation is when the two occur together. Both kinds of stress shut off hormone production and interfere with thyroid function on their own. Together, they are a vicious force that spirals in on itself. Stress begets stress, which begets stress, which begets stress.

Unfortunately, this is a common phenomenon in the Western world. Not only are most of us stressed out in general, but some fairly nasty ideas about body image and food plague the American psyche and make it that much harder for women to escape the trap of restrictive behavior.

Body image issues, negative self-esteem, and a culture obsessed with appearance and thinness mean that millions of women and girls starve and doubt and hate themselves. Young female athletes are particularly at risk for the confluence of these two stressors. These athletes are so numerous, in fact, that they have a condition named after them: female athletic triad syndrome. The three elements of the triad are low body weight, excessive exercise, and limited eating (often related to body image issues). These factors combine to give women enough stress to lose their menstrual cycles and fertility. Other symptoms of female athletic triad syndrome include hair loss, cold hands and feet, fatigue, dry skin, low body weight, increased healing time for injuries, anemia, low blood pressure, and symptoms of low estrogen, such as increased incidence of bone fractures.

These symptoms are not limited to the young athletes who gave them their name. Physiological manifestations of punitive behavior and negative body image are common among women simply doing their best in the modern world. The most important tools for overcoming female athletic triad syndrome and all restrictive body image behaviors are acceptance, forgiveness, patience, and love, all of which are dealt with extensively in Step 5.

PCOS: the complex diagnosis

To receive an official PCOS diagnosis, you need to have two of the following three things: elevated male sex hormone levels, irregular menstrual periods, and multiple small cysts on your ovaries. Symptoms include acne, low libido, difficulty losing weight, male-pattern hair loss on the top of the head, and male-pattern hair growth on the face, arms, and back. We saw earlier how insulin resistance and testosterone can cause PCOS to develop, but that is only one part of the story.

In the majority of PCOS cases, the primary cause of hormone imbalance *is* insulin resistance. For this reason, medical professionals usually treat PCOS patients with insulin-sensitizing drugs or birth control pills, both of which can reduce testosterone levels. Patients are often told to lose weight and exercise more. However, a wide variety of other factors can cause the development of cystic ovaries, and if health professionals do not pay attention to them, women who do not fit neatly into the insulin resistance category will never receive the treatment they need.

More than being a condition of simple testosterone excess, PCOS is actually a condition of imbalance between male and female sex hormones. On one side of the spectrum, two primary factors increase male sex hormone levels: insulin gives rise to testosterone excess, and stress gives rise to DHEA-S excess. On the other side of the spectrum—the side that typically goes unnoticed by health professionals—reducing levels of the female sex hormones estrogen and progesterone in response to physiological and psychological stress also tips the scales in favor of male sex hormones.

A third cause of PCOS is birth control pills: progesterone, estrogen, testosterone, and other pituitary hormones can fall out of balance when a woman takes birth control pills. As a result, many women who go off the pill exhibit symptoms of PCOS and have trouble menstruating for a significant time, sometimes having to wait a whole year before the pituitary gland normalizes and hormones get back into proper form and balance.

A fourth cause of PCOS is hypothyroidism, which contributes to the growth of ovarian cysts. The fifth and final cause is poor gut flora health and leaky gut, which has been shown not only to disrupt health hormone production but also to increase inflammation and toxin load higher than many women's reproductive systems can handle. Given the number of factors, it's no surprise that millions of women struggle with ovarian cysts.

So many different things can cause PCOS. It is not the easy diagnosis that so many medical professionals would have us believe. Millions of women receive inadequate treatment because of the failure to recognize its complexity. Recommendations for overcoming PCOS should be sensitive to these differences and tailored to each woman's unique needs.

The role of hypothyroidism in infertility

The thyroid gland is important for reproductive function because it is responsible for getting energy to cells. Without sufficient energy, cells shut down and cannot do their jobs. As a result, many bodily functions falter. Reproductive cells in particular do not have the energy they need to perform their regular reproductive functions.

Hypothyroidism is a condition worth investigating and tackling with your doctor. Thyroid medication may be in order, depending on how severe the hypothyroidism is and whether you have Hashimoto's thyroiditis. Regardless, taking proper nutritional care of the thyroid gland can significantly boost fertility. For more on hypothyroidism and how to overcome it, see the section on hypothyroidism and energy on page 209.

The role of post–birth control syndrome in infertility

A final lifestyle contributor to infertility is hormonal birth control. When women stop using hormonal birth control, they sometimes experience difficulty regaining their menstrual cycles. The longer they report having been on birth control, I have noticed, the more likely they are to have trouble.

How and why does this happen? For one, putting external hormones into your bloodstream signals to your pituitary gland that you don't need to produce these hormones on your own. This is all well and good while you are on the pill. However, when you remove the external hormones from the equation, your pituitary gland might not leap back into action. All its work has been done for it for the last several years, so it might not remember quite how to send and receive signals properly. For another, these additional hormones may build up in your liver such that when you stop taking the pill, your liver continues to release the hormones into your bloodstream, "tricking" your body into thinking that you are still on the pill.

I have worked with women who, after quitting the pill, have taken a year or more to resume cycling. The best thing to do in this situation is to eat a nourishing a diet rich in vitamins and minerals, support healthy insulin signaling and metabolic health, support gut health by eliminating gut irritants and consuming probiotic foods, and make sure that you are as relaxed as possible.

A brief note on pregnancy

Much as I would love to help you overcome the many woes of pregnancy in the modern world, I could not find a way to do it justice without doubling the size of this book. Fortunately, there are a myriad of helpful books devoted to natural pregnancy and childbirth, some of which are listed at the end of the book under "Resources for Further Reading."

Taking liver-supporting supplements such as milk thistle extract may also help. With nourishment as your top priority, your body will receive the resources it needs to support healthy hormone production and can resume cycling on its own.

What to do for infertility and irregular menstrual cycles:

○ Work with your doctor to rule out physiological problems such as fallopian tube irregularities.

○ Get your hormone levels tested. This will tell you broadly which category of infertility you fall into. Testosterone, estrogen, progesterone, prolactin, LH, FSH, and DHEA-S are crucial hormones to test in order to understand how your menstrual cycle might be dysregulated. Elevated testosterone and DHEA-S, plus an elevation of FSH over LH, are typical hormone profiles of PCOS. Low estrogen, progesterone, LH, and FSH are typical of stress-based infertility and female athletic triad syndrome. High DHEA-S indicates stress and pregnenolone steal. Abnormal TSH, T3, and T4 indicate various thyroid problems, which can be key players in all aspects of infertility.

○ Accept the uniqueness of your situation and any complexities that arise. No two women are alike, so each case of infertility will manifest itself differently. It is likely that many different components are part of your problem—for example, both insulin resistance and a history of dieting and stress.

○ In consultation with your doctor, consider addressing symptoms with medicinal treatments, such as birth control pills, hormone replacement therapy, insulin-sensitizing drugs, or thyroid hormone replacement. While these treatments are not long-term solutions, they can support reproductive health as you work on bolstering your natural health.

○ Using the natural remedies outlined in this book, begin working on the problems that are contributing to your infertility, such as stress, starvation, or insulin resistance. Modify your diet and lifestyle to meet your specific needs.

○ If you are insulin resistant, eat an anti-inflammatory, gut-healing diet with low to moderate amounts of fruits and starches.

○ If you have hypothyroidism, work to overcome it by using the methods described in the section on energy (see page 209).

○ If you exercise excessively, have a history of dieting, or restrict your food intake, eat more at each meal, and eat more meals. Make sure to eat at least 100 grams of carbohydrate every day—a few servings of fruit or potato plus ample vegetables.

○ Eat a minimum of 50 grams of fat each day to support hormone production.

○ Consider therapy to soothe the effects of stress on your reproductive system.

○ For PCOS, consider supplementing with magnesium, zinc, and chromium to improve insulin sensitivity. Vitamin D and calcium have also been shown to improve ovarian function. B vitamins are particularly helpful for clearing homocysteine, a molecule that has been tied to PCOS, out of the blood.

○ Support adrenal health with magnesium, B vitamins, and vitamin C.

○ Increase the amount of positive romantic and sexual activity in your life, which can help boost reproductive hormone production.

Family Planning:
Be protected

One of the biggest issues facing women of reproductive age is pregnancy prevention. Do you go on the pill? Maybe. What are the effects? Variable. Will the pill hurt your fertility in the long run? Possibly. Are there different options? Too many. How can you have the most natural and easy sex life? No one is sure. Is a natural and easy sex life even possible? Yes!

Birth control may seem insurmountably complex, but in reality it is quite simple. It can be broken down into two broad categories: hormonal and non-hormonal. Non-hormonal birth control is hormonally safer and more natural. But that doesn't rule out hormonal options. As a natural woman, you can still find a hormonal method that works for you. It is a matter of making the best choice possible given the benefits and drawbacks of each method. Each one has a long list of pros and cons.

Sexually transmitted infections

Unfortunately, there are no natural remedies for STIs such as gonorrhea, chlamydia, syphilis, herpes, HPV, and HIV. In addition to receiving clinical treatment, the best thing you can do naturally to support your body in overcoming or mitigating these problems is to support your immune system. Stress management, sleep, moderate exercise, sunlight or vitamin D supplementation, and an anti-inflammatory diet rich in greens, healthful animal products and organ meats, seafood, and natural carbohydrates are the best means by which to do so.

All birth control methods except the condom fail to prevent STIs; they prevent only pregnancy. So get tested, *both* of you!

How it works: hormonal birth control

Hormonal birth control disrupts the natural menstrual cycle and prevents ovulation from occurring. Ovulation is triggered by a hormone called luteinizing hormone, or LH, which is secreted by the pituitary gland. LH cannot be secreted if progesterone is present in the bloodstream. The whole idea of hormonal birth control, then, is to sufficiently elevate progesterone levels in the blood to prevent ovulation. Some formulations of the pill contain only progesterone. Others combine progesterone with estrogen. All of them contain hormones that are synthetic varieties, which are not identical to human hormones.

The primary drawbacks of hormonal birth control: side effects and risks

Side effects

Gynecologists often tell women that finding a birth control pill is just a matter of trying different formulas until one "works." The reason so many pills don't work for so many women, however, is that each woman has a uniquely designed reproductive system. The more you interfere with this system, the more damage you might do or risks you might incur. Some women go on the pill and do not suffer at all. In others, significant and unpleasant changes swiftly rear their ugly heads.

The general side effects of hormonal birth control include headaches, migraines, menstrual irregularities, spotting, nausea, vomiting, mood swings, insomnia, anxiety, depression, weight gain, acne, breast pain or tenderness, fatigue, and low libido. Importantly, one side effect of birth control that is not well known is its deleterious effect on gut flora. The birth control pill can deplete your healthy gut flora population, making you more susceptible to health issues beyond the standard birth control list.

Risks

Worse than the side effects for some women are the risks involved with hormonal birth control. There are three primary categories of risk. The first is drospirenone-related risk. Drospirenone is a compound found in several different birth control formulations that appeals to many women because it can block male hormone activity. This characteristic makes it popular for women who suffer from PCOS, acne, and other problems caused by excess testosterone. Yet drospirenone can also make the body create a potassium reserve. Excess potassium can lead to hyperkalemia, which can be fatal. As such, women on drospirenone-containing pills need to have their potassium levels checked regularly, as well as to be on the lookout for cardiovascular symptoms such as muscle weakness and heart palpitations. Moreover, users of drospirenone-containing pills may have a higher risk of blood clots than users of birth control pills that do not contain drospirenone. Drospirenone-containing pills include Yaz, Yazmin, Gianvi, Ocella, Syeda, Zarah, Beaz, and Safyral.

The second category of risk pertains to the complications of estrogen supplementation. Estrogen-containing formulations of birth control increase the risk of breast cancer, blood clots, thrombosis (painful and potentially harmful blood clotting), stroke, and heart attack. Young, perfectly healthy women have in fact suffered strokes and died, quite possibly because of the way their blood clotted from the pills they were taking.

The final major risk of hormonal birth control is that it can significantly and semi-permanently disrupt natural hormone production. As I explained in the section on infertility, inserting foreign hormones into the bloodstream causes the pituitary gland to adapt to those levels. It doesn't need—or even want—to produce hormones if it doesn't have to.

When you go off of hormonal birth control, your pituitary gland might not jump back into action the way you'd like it to. It is also possible that excess estrogen has built up in your liver and will continue to flow through your bloodstream for several months after you stop taking the pill—which extends the amount of time you are hormonally prevented from ovulating. Many women have no problem transitioning to life post–birth control, but others do have problems. For those of us hoping to have babies after getting off the pill, this is a real concern. Healing can take several months if not years.

Being on hormonal birth control can also mask underlying hormone problems. Many women go on the pill in adolescence and then, when they stop taking it, start exhibiting symptoms of PCOS, PMS, and other menstrual disorders. The longer these problems go untreated, the harder they are to overcome. Because of these hormone-disrupting and masking effects, as well as the risks and side effects, many women choose to steer clear of hormonal birth control options.

Hormonal options

The pill

The pill is the most common form of birth control. Up to 80 percent of women of reproductive age have taken birth control pills at some point in their lives.[29] This is an enormous number! Some women are on progesterone-only pills, and others take estrogen-progesterone combinations.

Estrogen was added to the pill after it was invented to mitigate spotting as well as to help restore balance between estrogen and progesterone, which is necessary for clear skin, good sleep, and mental health. However, some (arguably most) women in the Western world don't need more estrogen.

Birth control pills generally induce a period in order to help a woman "stay regular." It is healthy to menstruate at least a few times a year. Menstruation clears up the reproductive organs and lowers the risk of cancer developing on ovarian tissue. Beyond those few times, however, the reason pills induce monthly periods is largely psychological: the pharmaceutical companies that designed the pill thought women would be more comfortable on the pill if they still menstruated once a month. Many women responded by telling them that that was a joke, so later formulations began inducing menstrual periods once every three, four, or even six months. They induce menstruation by replacing hormonal pills with sugar placebos for up to one week. This change reduces the amount of progesterone in the blood, which is the body's natural signal to menstruate.

Some pills contain more hormones than others. Dozens of varieties exist. The drawback of the pill is that it is one of the most hormonal methods of birth control. It has potential to cause significant changes in a woman's life, both in the short term with respect to symptoms and in the long term with respect to hormonal shifts and pituitary function.

The implant (Implanon)

The implant is a small, progesterone-leaching rod that a physician inserts on the underside of a woman's arm. The implant steadily releases small doses of progesterone into the body. Once inserted, it is effective for up to three years.

Because the implant supplies a continual dosage of progesterone, it does not induce a regular cycle the way most other birth control methods do. For the majority of women on the implant, periods become light but unpredictable. For roughly 30 percent of women, menstruation stops completely within one year of use.

The shot (Depo Provera)

The shot is a relatively high-dose progesterone injection that a physician administers once every three months. This method of birth control has one of the highest success rates, as it leaves very little room for human error, and it has the additional benefit of being hassle-free. On the other hand, in order for the progesterone to be effective for three months, the shot delivers a fairly high dose, which can be problematic for hormone balance for some women.

The patch (Ortho Evra)

The patch is a progesterone-estrogen combination. The small, beige, sticky patch is applied anywhere on the skin and is replaced weekly. It generates much higher levels of estrogen in the blood than the pharmaceutical company had anticipated, however. This results in a greater risk of blood clots—and shortly after the patch was released, lawsuits began mounting. In 2005, under an agreement with the FDA, Ortho Evra added a black-box warning to its package stating that patch users are exposed to roughly 60 percent more estrogen than the typical pill user, resulting in an "approximate doubling of risk of serious blood clots."

Yet women who suffer from low estrogen levels may benefit greatly from estrogen input. The appropriate amount of estrogen varies by individual, so it is worth discussing these issues with your doctor if you are interested in how much estrogen you should (be daring to) take.

The vaginal ring (NuvaRing)

The NuvaRing is a flexible plastic ring that is inserted into the vagina once a month. It was instantly popular upon release because it offers an easy contraception method with a lower risk of blood clots than the patch. The NuvaRing is also a combination method, yet it contains less estrogen than both the patch and combination pills.

Many women believe that the NuvaRing is a gentler form of birth control—that it won't cause hormonal disturbances—because it sits in the vagina and therefore acts *locally* rather than universally in the body, supposedly mitigating the side effects. But I have yet to find any evidence that this is the case. If anything, the real reason the NuvaRing may have fewer side effects than other methods is that it releases a lower dose of hormones into the blood.

The progesterone intrauterine device (IUD)

The final form of hormonal birth control is the progesterone intrauterine device (IUD). The IUD has become wildly popular— the most current estimate by the World Health Organization is that up to 160 million women worldwide use some form of the IUD.[30] An OB/GYN or other certified practitioner inserts the IUD into the uterus. This makes it similar to the implant, but the IUD lasts even longer, an average of five years.

The progesterone IUD is coated with a membrane that regulates the release of progesterone into the uterus. It releases levonorgestrel, a type of progesterone, at an initial rate of 20 micrograms per day, declining to a rate of 14 micrograms after five years. In comparison, birth control pills can contain as much as 150 micrograms of levonorgestrel, all of which feed right into the bloodstream. As such, the IUD offers the lowest possible dose of hormones out of hormonal birth control methods. It can be used for up to seven years.

How it works: non-hormonal birth control

The great benefit of non-hormonal birth control is that it is hormone free, which means that your natural hormones get to run the show. As a woman interested in natural health, this is probably an appealing option for you. Unfortunately there are not many non-hormonal options, though each of them has its own set of unique qualities that may suit your birth control needs.

Non-hormonal options

The copper IUD

The copper IUD has the same shape and implantation method as the progesterone IUD, but functions differently. Instead of interfering with hormone production, it acts as a spermicide within the uterus, making its failure rate quite low.

There is a drawback, however. Copper increases the amount of inflammatory molecules called *prostaglandins* and white blood cells within the uterine and tubal fluids, which can exacerbate any regular inflammation that occurs during the menstrual cycle. If you are sensitive to inflammation or have a painful menstrual cycle already, an IUD may make cramping and blood flow worse. On the other hand, with an anti-inflammatory diet and properly balanced hormones, you have the power to tame these effects.

The one potential threat of the copper IUD is copper toxicity, which is often underemphasized by medical professionals. If your body receives more copper than it can handle—particularly a risk if copper's counterbalance, zinc, is not supplemented or consumed in high quantities while using the IUD—you can experience crippling side effects. If you have a copper IUD, consider a zinc supplement to prevent copper toxicity.

Tubal ligation

Tubal ligation is the medical term for "getting your tubes tied." It is an outpatient procedure that comes with all the risks of infection and anesthesia that surgery always does, but no more. Tubal ligation is a mostly permanent procedure. It *can* be reversed in many cases—as many as 70 percent of reversals are successful. Nonetheless, the procedure cuts, plugs, or cauterizes the fallopian tubes, so it should not be undertaken unless you are certain that you are done having children.

Tubal ligation is an excellent choice for hormonal health. It has virtually no impact on natural hormone levels. In fact, menstruation continues to occur as it otherwise would in most women who undergo this procedure, since interfering with the fallopian tubes does not interfere with ovarian processes. The only way hormone health can be hurt is in the case of one rare side effect: decreased blood flow to reproductive tissue, which can lead to decreased hormone production.

The Fertility Awareness Method

The Fertility Awareness Method (FAM) may be the most controversial of all birth control methods. It is definitely the most natural, but it is also the riskiest. It depends on getting to know your body, predicting your fertile window, and then avoiding unprotected sex during that window.

The trick of the FAM is to identify the physiological markers of ovulation. These markers include spiking levels of luteinizing hormone (LH) in the blood, elevated basal body temperature 24 hours after ovulation, thickened and increased volume of vaginal discharge, heightened libido, and the cervix moving upward in the body. Many methods and tools can be used to track these changes; I have included a guide to FAM in the "Resources for Further Reading" list at the end of the book.

You may be skeptical that these markers are accurate, or you may worry that you will read a signal incorrectly. Taken together, however, the signals yield powerful evidence of ovulation (given that you ovulate regularly). As you become more accustomed to this method, you will become more familiar with the shapes of these feelings and fluctuations and become more accurate with your predictions.

Ovulation lasts for approximately 36 hours. Is this the only time you have to avoid unprotected sex? Hardly! Sperm can survive in the reproductive cavity for up to seven days. This means that with FAM, you must avoid having sex during the week preceding and in the week following ovulation, which divides your sex life neatly in half. For approximately two weeks each month you can have unprotected sex, and during the other two weeks you must abstain or use prophylactics.

Your chances of getting pregnant

A perfectly fertile and healthy couple has a 1 in 4 or 1 in 5 chance of conceiving during the woman's fertile period. This means that the vast majority of couples trying to conceive will do so within a year.

Libido:
Be ravenous

According to a study published in the *Journal of the American Medical Association,* approximately 43 percent of women (compared to 31 percent of men) suffer from low libido for one reason or another.[31] Strikingly, this number is thought to underestimate the real level of sexual dysfunction in the U.S.

How it works: libido

Like all other issues of reproductive health, having a healthy libido is all about hormone balance. Testosterone needs to be pumping, but not in excess. Estrogen needs to be present, but cannot be dominant. Progesterone is crucial. All three of these hormones play excitatory roles in the brain. They work in complex harmony with neurotransmitters such as dopamine and must be present in proper balance.

Because of this need for balance, all the hormone imbalances discussed in this book, such as PCOS, hypothalamic amenorrhea, female athletic triad syndrome, post–birth control pill syndrome, and menopause, can cause of low libido. Troubleshooting low libido is by and large a matter of figuring out what kind of hormone imbalance you suffer from and then mitigating that problem.

Neurotransmitters are chemicals such as serotonin and dopamine that transmit signals in the brain. They are largely responsible for just about every craving, feeling, and brain state, so supporting optimal neurotransmitter function and balance is crucial.

Libido and your heart and brain

There are many ways in which your psychological self can interrupt your sex life, and you may not even be aware of them. How do things go awry? The reasons are nearly infinite. Perhaps your libido has been quashed by a negative sexual experience. Or perhaps you are too stressed out by other factors to care about sex, or relations between you and your partner are strained. Perhaps your lover is a mean, ugly lump. Perhaps you are frustrated with your partner, feel rejected, or do not feel properly loved and safe in the bedroom.

Many of those factors fall outside my realm of expertise, largely because they deal with interpersonal relationships. Aside from needing to have good relationships with the people with whom you are sexual, however, a fierce libido requires that you have a good relationship with your own sexuality. Truly believing that you are sexy is one of the greatest boons for a healthy libido. Being at home in your body and loving your sexual self are virtual prerequisites to a good sex life. Experiencing sex positively and embracing it as not just a natural but also an empowering and joyful part of life can't hurt, either. This is the stuff on which the *Sexy by Nature* paradigm thrives. Need help feeling sexy and empowered and loving yourself? Dive into Step 5.

The dominant kinds of hormone imbalance are:

○ Too much testosterone, which is usually a result of high insulin levels in the blood.

○ Too little progesterone, which is usually a result of stress.

○ Too little estrogen, which can be a result of low body weight, weight loss, dieting, ovarian malfunction, or stress.

○ Too much estrogen relative to progesterone, which can be a result of consuming phytoestrogens such as flax and soy, being overweight, being stressed, taking birth control pills, or not exercising enough.

Low dopamine and low serotonin can also cause low libido. Dopamine is the most important neurotransmitter for sexual prowess and reproductive function.

What to do for a ravenous libido

○ Reduce your consumption of sugar-rich foods for insulin sensitivity.

○ Consume a diet low in phytoestrogens such as soy and flax to help rebalance estrogen and progesterone levels.

○ Consider adding phytoestrogens such as soy and flax to your diet on occasion to see if they boost your libido, which is possible based on the way your body processes phytoestrogens.

○ Eat an anti-inflammatory, nutrient-rich, gut-healing diet such as the *Sexy by Nature* diet.

○ Consume at least 50 grams of fat each day to support healthy hormone production.

○ Reduce stress.

○ Exercise to increase dopamine levels; almost nothing increases dopamine levels as well as exercise does.

○ Increase serotonin production by consuming adequate protein (at least 50 grams), getting adequate sun exposure, consuming at least a few servings of natural carbohydrates each day, and, perhaps most important of all, sleeping deeply.

○ Cultivate communication, mutual respect, and love with your partner(s).

○ Develop a positive relationship with your body and your sexuality.

○ Fake it 'til you make it: have sex! Even in the lowest lows of my hormone deficiencies, I felt my struggling libido bounce back in the weeks following romantic and sexual encounters. I should not have been so surprised, because sex has potent dopamine-releasing effects.

○ Get lovey. Romantic feelings stimulate dopamine and serotonin production, as well as the release of sex hormones such as estrogen.

Cramps:
Be pain-free

Though we often associate menstrual cramps with PMS, they are actually a separate phenomenon. What causes cramps, and how can you overcome them?

How it works: menstrual cramps

Nutrient deficiencies, inflammation, and hormone imbalance are the primary causes of cramping. They are also often the culprits in heavy menstrual flow, so you may be able to kill two birds with one stone by addressing menstrual cramping.

Certain nutrients are key components in the contraction and relaxation of muscle tissue. Electrolytes in particular, which include potassium, calcium, sodium, and magnesium, have well-known muscle-relaxing effects. A deficiency in any of these nutrients is a common cause of muscle cramping everywhere in the body. This is especially true of magnesium for menstrual cramping. Magnesium is responsible for the relaxation of muscle tissue. Without magnesium, the muscles around your uterus cannot release tension.

During the menstrual cycle, reproductive tissue contracts and secretes inflammatory molecules. This process is perfectly safe and healthy if it occurs in a body with a healthy and smooth-running immune system. If you have any kind of systemic inflammation, however, or your immune system is in panic mode as a result of diet and lifestyle choices, you may experience an extreme amount of cramping.

The final and most important piece of this puzzle is hormone balance. The type of hormone imbalance that leads to cramping is called *estrogen dominance*. When you have too much estrogen relative to progesterone in your body, the lining of your uterus becomes unusually thick. With a thicker lining, you have an increased amount of tissue from which inflammatory molecules can be secreted. A thicker uterine lining also means that more tissue needs to be shed, so during menstruation you have to squeeze more material through a small space. You also end up bleeding more for the sheer fact of having to shed more material.

On the Standard American Diet, it is easy to have all three of these problems. Nutrient deficiencies, inflammation, and estrogen dominance abound. Nearly infinite food choices can exacerbate these problems over time. It's no wonder menstruation gets such a bad rap in the modern world. Fortunately, the women I have worked with on reducing inflammation and correcting hormone balance have reported reduced cramping, reduced PMS symptoms, and lighter and shorter menstrual periods after switching to the *Sexy by Nature* diet. If that's not motivation enough to adopt this diet, I don't know what is.

Estrogen dominance

Estrogen dominance is one of the primary causes of PMS, but that is not its only drawback. Symptoms associated with estrogen dominance include being overweight, weight gain, mood swings, emotional sensitivity, heavy periods, breast tenderness, headaches, decreased libido, sluggish metabolism, and insomnia. Conditions that are found more often in women with estrogen dominance and that may develop explicitly as a result of it include cystic fibroids, endometriosis, adenomyosis, hypothyroidism, breast cancer, cervical cancer, and ovarian cancer. From the list of symptoms and associated diseases, it's a no-brainer that estrogen dominance is a problem that deserves attention.

Estrogen dominance plagues millions of women, perhaps more so than any other hormone imbalance discussed in this book. This is largely because estrogen is produced in fat cells, and the majority of American women are overweight. But that's not the only way to develop estrogen dominance. Causes of estrogen dominance are both powerful and diverse and include:

○ **Being overweight:** Fat cells perform a function called *aromatization* that converts testosterone to estrogen. The more body fat you have, the more estrogen your body produces.

○ **Overburdening the liver:** The liver is responsible for clearing the body of old hormones, especially estrogen. If the liver is overburdened by a hyper-caloric, inflammatory diet that includes high volumes of sugar, alcohol, processing chemicals, and toxins, it becomes sluggish in its ability to process hormones.

○ **Being stressed:** Stress decreases the production of progesterone in the body. When progesterone levels decline relative to estrogen, symptoms of estrogen dominance emerge.

○ **Consuming phyto- and xenoestrogens:** Consuming estrogens from toxic chemicals such as fertilizers found on industrial produce and BPA is unquestionably a bad idea. Consuming plant estrogens such as soy and flax may be helpful sometimes, but in the case of estrogen dominance, it probably is not.

○ **Eating a low-fiber diet:** Estrogen is processed not only in the liver but also by gut flora, and it is excreted through the digestive track. Many other variables are likely at play here, but the general idea is that estrogen can be reabsorbed through the intestinal walls. If you do not eat any fiber, and you therefore have little added bulk to your stool, your digestive process will slow down. When it takes a long time for your body to excrete waste, estrogen sits in the gut for too long and is reabsorbed into the bloodstream. Fiber may help speed the digestive process along and keep the estrogen moving. Fiber supplements are unnecessary, however. The fiber you get from natural fruits and vegetables in the *Sexy by Nature* diet is plenty.

○ **Poor gut flora:** Since having poor gut flora is another way to slow down digestion and impair estrogen processing, it is another means by which estrogen levels rise.

○ **Taking the pill:** Sometimes birth control pills help decrease estrogen levels. Other times, the pill elevates estrogen levels above progesterone significantly enough to cause extreme discomfort.

○ **Living a sedentary lifestyle:** Exercise improves insulin sensitivity, liver function, weight loss, and stress reduction.

Estrogen dominance has many causes and may seem too complicated to overcome easily, but by emphasizing exercise, phytoestrogen moderation, and anti-inflammatory, gut-enriching, liver-supporting foods, the *Sexy by Nature* approach to health addresses all of them in one fell swoop.

Endometriosis

Cramps are made worse by a condition known as *endometriosis*, which affects nearly 5 million women in the United States.[32] Endometriosis is characterized by the implantation of endometrial tissue outside its normal locations. This tissue can go virtually anywhere it wants in the abdominal cavity, but it usually sticks near the reproductive organs. Throughout the menstrual cycle, this tissue acts as though it were a part of the normal menstrual package. It becomes inflamed, swells, and bleeds just like normal endometrial tissue.

Having endometriosis can radically compound the pain you experience during your menstrual cycle and increase the number of locations in which you feel it. Unfortunately, endometrial tissue does not go away once it has been implanted. It can, however, be soothed and reduced by an anti-inflammatory diet that includes an adequate intake of omega-3 fat, magnesium supplementation, stress reduction, sleep, and exercise. You can also prevent it by supporting the immune system. The reason these tissues get implanted in the first place is usually that the immune system isn't strong enough to fight them off. Adequate sun exposure, vitamin D, sleep, and a diet rich in vitamins and minerals like the *Sexy by Nature* diet are supremely helpful in supporting immune function and preventing endometriosis.

What to do for cramping

○ Eliminate or minimize your consumption of omega-6 oils to reduce inflammation.

○ Eliminate sugars, particularly around the time of the month, to prevent inflammatory blood sugar spikes.

○ Eliminate gut-irritating foods such as grains, legumes, and dairy.

○ Reduce estrogen dominance by the methods listed above: reduce stress, eat an anti-inflammatory diet like the *Sexy by Nature* diet, consume plenty of vegetables and fiber, support liver health by reducing toxin load and focusing on natural foods, and avoid phytoestrogens such as soy and flax.

○ Consume leafy greens, which contain high amounts of an enzyme that helps the liver clear estrogen out of the bloodstream.

○ Consider adding vitamin E to your diet or following a supplementation regimen. Vitamin E by itself has been shown to reduce pain from cramping, possibly because of its antioxidant and anti-inflammatory effects. Good sources of vitamin E are leafy green vegetables, peppers, asparagus, tomatoes, carrots, almonds, and meat products, especially grass-fed beef.

○ Supplement with cod liver oil or fish oil, or eat a couple of servings of fatty fish such as salmon every week to counteract inflammation.

○ Eat a diet rich in magnesium. Leafy green vegetables, halibut, nuts, and chocolate are all good magnesium foods.

○ Consider supplementing with at least 400 milligrams of magnesium a day, particularly around the time of the month.

○ Consider supplements that may help with estrogen detox and liver health, such as milk thistle extract, alpha lipoic acid, and the amino acid N-acetylcysteine (NAC).

PMS:
Be calm

In some ways, being a woman is uniquely challenging. Throughout the course of a regular month, we bleed out of our vaginas for a week, we enjoy one week of peace and freedom, and then we ovulate and have two weeks of fluctuating estrogen and progesterone levels, which can lead to breast tenderness, water retention, acne, insomnia, moodiness, depression, anxiety, headaches, cravings, and cramping. Technically, you will only be diagnosed with PMS if you experience the mental symptoms, which include depression, irritability, anxiety, and mood swings. But the physical symptoms that accompany these are often equally unpleasant. What gives? Is menstruation supposed to be this way? Does it *have* to be this way?

How it works:
premenstrual syndrome

Menstruation is *not* supposed to be this way. It is not supposed to be painful, make you crazy, or make you depressed. Sure, even after you adopt a diet based on whole, natural foods, you may experience echoes of these symptoms. But you can greatly mitigate them by supporting the health of your reproductive and nervous systems. You have the power to turn what may be a truly terrible state into a mere inconvenience.

As far as theorists can tell, PMS is caused primarily by two things: estrogen dominance and neurotransmitter dysfunction.

Symptoms of estrogen dominance occur for many women in the two weeks prior to menstruation. In these two weeks, the body is gearing up for menstruation, so deviation from natural health and hormone balance is a fair bit easier than at other times of the month. Elevating estrogen over progesterone causes symptoms of PMS because the brain is full of receptors for these two hormones. When the brain encounters a hormone imbalance during this time, it has trouble achieving the level of stability it attains at other times of the month. Improper hormone balance can cause a decrease in serotonin, dopamine, and endorphin levels, all of which are important for mental health. Anxiety, irritability, depression, and insomnia may ensue. Correcting hormone balance is a primary concern for any woman experiencing trouble with PMS.

Maintaining neurotransmitter health is also crucial for avoiding PMS. Poor diet leads to poor neurotransmitter synthesis. Dietary elements particularly important for neurotransmitter synthesis are complete proteins—so make sure to eat sufficient protein throughout the day—vitamin C, and B vitamins, especially B_6. These nutrients are easily obtained from a diet rich in vegetables and animal products such as the *Sexy by Nature* diet, though supplementation might also be appropriate.

* * *

In addition to mitigating these two causes of PMS, you can support your mental health throughout the menstrual cycle by reducing inflammation, which can be a great help to your brain. Two of the most important ways to do so are by maintaining a healthy blood sugar metabolism—which helps neurotransmitters function more stably—and focusing on omega-3 fat.

Omega-3 fat is a great tool for fighting PMS not only because it is anti-inflammatory, but also because the brain is composed largely of fat. The higher-quality fat you have in your diet, the higher-quality brain function you are going to have. Omega-3 fat helps with the flexibility of neuronal structures, which ultimately leads to greater peace and alleviation of PMS symptoms.

PMDD

Premenstrual dysphoric disorder (PMDD) is a more severe form of PMS that affects between 3 and 8 percent of American women.[33] Instead of being a nuisance that turns you into a cranky toad for a week like PMS can, PMDD is debilitating. It is usually characterized by extreme depression, sadness, despair, tension, anxiety, panic attacks, extreme sensitivity to emotional situations, uncontrollable crying, apathy, extreme and/or chronic fatigue, binge eating, and severe headaches. Women who suffer from PMDD demonstrate with much more statistical strength a deficiency in the function of estrogen receptors in the brain. PMDD is often treated with SSRIs and other antidepressants, though the same interventions used for PMS can provide some relief for PMDD.

What to do for PMS

○ Exercise, which increases serotonin and dopamine levels.

○ Get adequate sleep to raise serotonin levels.

○ Reduce estrogen dominance by the methods listed above: reduce stress, eat an anti-inflammatory diet that eschews the potential gut irritants grains, legumes, and dairy, consume plenty of vegetables and fiber, and support liver health by reducing toxin load and focusing on natural foods. Leafy greens are particularly helpful since they have potent liver-supporting effects.

○ Consider supplements that may help with estrogen detox, such as milk thistle extract, alpha lipoic acid, and the amino acid N-acetylcysteine (NAC).

○ Eliminate phytoestrogens such as soy and flax from your diet, and minimize exposure to xenoestrogens such as BPA (found in plastics) and fertilizers on the skins of fruits and vegetables.

○ Consume at least 50 grams of protein each day.

○ Eliminate or minimize omega-6 seed oil consumption and consume at least three servings of fatty fish such as salmon every week to reduce inflammation.

○ Consider supplementing with cod liver oil or a high-quality fish oil for omega-3 fat.

○ Eat animal products and vegetables for vitamins B and C, respectively, which support neurotransmitter synthesis.

○ Consider supplementing with 400 milligrams of magnesium daily to minimize anxiety, insomnia, and depression.

○ Expose yourself to the sun for 20 minutes every day, or consider supplementing with 2,000 to 5,000 IUD of vitamin D daily to provide crucial support for mental health.

Mental Health:
Be happy

One of the most important principles of *Sexy by Nature* is that psychological and physiological health are intrinsically linked. You cannot have one without the other. Happiness does not exist without sufficient neurotransmitter supply, for example. Nor will you have healthy adrenal glands if you do not feel positive and hopeful.

The psychological basis of mental health is very real, and is best handled with therapy, love, and attentive self-care. There is also a significant physiological component of mental health. Unfortunately, I do not have the room or the expertise to give the physiological basis of mental health the attention it deserves here. Nonetheless, I can speak broadly about the importance of nutrition for supporting a healthy mental life, and I can urge you to be aware of and care for your mental health in this journey in the same way that you care for your physical health.

If you find that you struggle with depression and/or anxiety no matter how much psychological healing you do, there may be an underlying physiological cause that can be addressed first with a diet that focuses on whole, nourishing foods, and second with the help of a medical professional who can help you figure out and address your specific needs within this paradigm.

How it works: anxiety and depression

The causes of depression and anxiety for women, because they are rooted in endocrine and neurological health, are quite similar to the causes of PMS. Hormone imbalance, inflammation, poor neurotransmitter production and maintenance, poor gut health, inadequate brain support, nutrient deficiencies, and sedentariness can all contribute to poor mental health. There are many other factors, myriads of them, and all quite complicated, too, but the ones listed here can at least be supported by a commitment to the nourishing principles of the *Sexy by Nature* diet.

What to do for anxiety and depression

○ Consult a physician first and foremost.

○ Reach out to and garner the support of family and friends.

○ Consult a psychologist or engage other therapy methods.

○ Balance hormone levels however you need to. If you are estrogen dominant, follow the prescriptions for estrogen dominance: reduce stress, eat an anti-inflammatory diet like the *Sexy by Nature* diet, consume plenty of vegetables and fiber, support liver health by reducing toxin load and focusing on natural foods, and avoid phytoestrogens such as soy and flax. If you are low on reproductive hormones, focus on reducing physical and psychological stress.

○ Consume fatty fish such as salmon several times a week, or supplement with cod liver oil or a high-quality fish oil. This is one of the more well-studied and effective natural methods of soothing depression and mental health disturbances.

○ Eliminate sugar and processed foods to reduce blood sugar spikes and keep insulin levels steady.

○ Eliminate omega-6 seed oils to reduce inflammation in the brain.

○ Eliminate gut-irritating and inflammatory foods such as grains, legumes, and dairy.

o Support neurotransmitter health with a diet of complete and sufficient protein, animal products for B vitamins, and vegetables and fruits for vitamin C.

o Include at least 100 grams of carbohydrate (a few servings of fruit or starchy vegetables) in your diet per day to support serotonin production.

o Increase the quality and duration of sleep.

o Reduce stress as much as possible.

o Support healthy gut flora, which are crucial for mental health, with probiotics or by consuming fermented foods.

o Supplement with at least 400 milligrams of magnesium a day, which can be particularly helpful for anxiety and depression.

o Exercise to increase serotonin and dopamine levels. Exercise has been shown to be at least as effective as antidepressants at mitigating depression, if not more so.[34]

5: Strut

"I am so beautiful, sometimes people weep when they see me. And it has nothing to do with what I look like really, it is just that I gave myself the power to say that I am beautiful, and if I could do that, maybe there is hope for them too. And the great divide between the beautiful and the ugly will cease to be. Because we are all what we choose."

—MARGARET CHO

The goal of this book is to empower you. It is to light a fire deep in your spirit. It is to give you the tools you need to nourish your body, make your body healthier, and come into a positive relationship with your body. My ultimate goal is to guide you into the thrill and excitement of being the woman inside it.

At the beginning of this book, I promised to show you how. Much of that work has now been done. In Step 1, the standard rules for health became old news. Control went out, and nature came in. Norms, restriction, punishment, mindless subjugation to authority, and a lack of appreciation for the complex healing power and beauty of the female body make it impossible to achieve real health. Stepping outside that game and writing our own rules enables us to take lessons from nature and provide our bodies with the support, love, and nourishment they need to repair themselves.

In Steps 2, 3, and 4, I provided you with detailed information about how the female body works so you can use that information to heal yourself. Your body does not need to be restricted or deprived in order to be healthy. It needs only to be given natural nourishment, with toxins kept to a minimum. Armed with these tools on the road to exultant health...now this is where the fun begins.

Self-love, self-determined sex appeal, and fearlessness are the trifecta—the three key players in empowered and sexy womanhood. Learning to embrace and to practice them in tandem with the *Sexy by Nature* dietary principles rounds out your health journey. You can be more than physically healthy. You can be ecstatic. You can feel sexy. And you can be excited to be in the skin you're in. Step 5 takes you all the way to self-loving sex goddess and empowers you to stay there for good—as a joyful, embodied woman and a brilliant light for others to follow.

Self-Love

No book on womanhood would be valid if it didn't address self-love. Very few of us have it, and just about everybody wants it. Though heartbreaking, this probably comes as no surprise. Loving ourselves is an enormous challenge in a culture full of competition, fear, and negativity. Yet without self-love, it is nearly impossible to be happy, to succeed, to treat yourself well, to treat others well, or to eat and live healthfully. Self-love is also crucial for being sexy. You cannot genuinely feel sexy without self-love supporting you from the ground up.

Loving myself was the bedrock of all the attitude shifts that I describe in this book. The acts of acceptance, forgiveness, and patience described in Step 1 are manifestations of love, and they are crucial to developing a life of health and happiness. The more I love myself, the more I accept myself as I am. And the more I can forgive what happened in the past and what may happen in the future, the more patience I have for myself and my body.

First in this chapter I lay out all the different ways in which you can love yourself, and then I provide concrete tools for cultivating these kinds of self-love. If I and thousands of other women can walk this walk, as Herculean a task as it may seem, trust me when I say that you can, too. Remember, this is not a journey about being hard on yourself and despairing when you cannot achieve perfection. It is about starting from square one with a positive attitude and learning to believe in and champion yourself over time.

Self-love and nature

If this book is about sexiness and nature, why am I talking about self-love? Does it seem a bit out of place? Like I said, no book about womanhood is complete without self-love, for one. Here are a few other reasons to include it:

Society has robbed us of our inherent, natural worth. This is a dramatic statement, but I stand by it. Objectification and sexism have put significant detrimental stamps on the female psyche. Yes, men struggle with self-love, too—just not in the same way that women do. Being the subjugated gender has done its damage. Fortunately, it is reversible. Stepping outside of social norms and paying better attention to what is natural helps us heal.

Nature says that we are all equally worthy and equally human. When you look at human DNA, you can't tell one person from another. Nature says that we are all human. We are all fallible. And therefore we all must be forgiven. If we weren't, society would be a hot mess of desperate and sad human beings.

Nature says there is no standard of beauty or goodness that we must live up to. Nature does not set norms. Nature does not tell us how to look or act. But nature has been trampled on in the rat race. Returning to natural principles enables us to appreciate ourselves exactly as we are and to love ourselves as unique women. It empowers us to love ourselves as natural beings and to let slide all the pressure demanding that we transform ourselves into an unnatural shape that would do us more harm than good.

Loving your physical self

When we women start trying to love ourselves, we come up against two different types of things to love: physical things and non-physical things.

The relationship between these two types of things is complicated, and our culture is pretty bad at drawing the distinction.

One example of this failure is the Dove Campaign for Real Beauty. Dove, a brand of toiletries, encourages women to "love the skin you're in" and stop trying to fit into society's ridiculous body standards. I approve. However, as powerful as this campaign may be, it may put too much emphasis on looks as a factor in self-love. "Love the skin you're in," the campaign says. It does not mention brains or personality or spirit. The marketers at Dove and many others claim that these ads empower women, but they do so only in the realm of physicality. Is physicality a bad thing? I don't think so, though I don't think it's entirely good, either.

Physical self-love is useful to many of the self-loving women I have encountered in my life. I am always curious about where their positivity comes from, so I often ask: Is it all about looks, or is it about something else? A lot of these women emphasize other things, like personality and smarts. Yet one woman I know, Mary, is serious about loving her physical body. She looks in the mirror every day and showers her curves with love. She caresses her voluptuous body, winks at herself, and says things like, "Hey, good lookin', you're awfully sexy today!"

This ritual helps Mary feel empowered in her body. It works for her. It makes her feel sexy, and it helps her love herself exactly as she is at that moment. The potential problem here—a problem that I still wrestle with myself—is that her self-love could get tied to her physical attributes. What then? What if she ties her self-love to her hourglass figure or her muscled calves? Disaster might strike if she becomes obsessed with specific body parts always being attractive or fit. Moreover, she might become overly invested in how she looks and lose sight of the larger picture.

My answer to these problems is to love my physical body without being married to its precise dimensions or character. I love it first and foremost because it gives me life, and only secondarily because of its unique shape and design. I forbid myself to love it because it fits some norm or ideal.

You must love your body, but you must also be flexible about what it looks like. Over the years, it is going to change a lot. Pregnancy, nursing, menopause, physical activities or injuries...all these ex-periences create powerful and unavoidable shifts in the shape of your body. So take it day by day. Appreciate your body as it is today. Love it for the hardships it has endured and the healing it is doing at this very moment. You do not have to be perfect. You do not have to adhere to a specific ideal that you or anyone else has set. You are you, and your body as it is *today* is just one part of that.

Love your physical body because it is short, or tall, or curvy, or not. Love it because it is dark-skinned or fair-skinned or olive-skinned or what-have-you. Love it because it has given you luscious red locks or earthy brown tresses. Celebrate its unique traits, but don't marry yourself to specific characteristics that might change over time. Love your body above all else because it is *yours,* and because it is feminine and lovely and you.

Loving your non-physical self

While loving your physicality can help you maintain a healthy relationship with your body, it must always come in the context of the wider whole. We are physical bodies, absolutely, but there is so much rich complexity to that fabric. We are smart, funny, warm, resourceful, and millions of other things to boot.

Being excited to be in your own skin is about more than your skin. It's about you. It is about your skills, your talents, your per-sonality, your charm. You are a package of millions of different at-tributes that are worthy of love. What is unique about you? What makes you tick? What makes you the delightful little corner of the universe that you are?

One of the best games to play is "What things are there to love about me?" I play it all the time. Sit down and think about the things there are to love about you. Be methodical. Try to think of everything everyone has ever said to you, every relationship you have had, and all the gifts your presence has bestowed on others. What comes up on your list?

An even better game to play is "Tell me what there is to love about me." It may sound ridiculous, or too difficult even to contemplate doing. But it's not. It's a simple act of honest communication. Sit down with a good friend, a family member, or your significant other and ask them why they love you. Don't be afraid of what they are going to say. Approach someone who is understanding and will be open to communicating with you. Explain that you are in the process of learning how to love yourself and that you're looking for some concrete things to focus on as you move forward. Say, "I know this may sound strange, but it would be helpful for me if you could share with me some reasons why you love me." Write them down together, or afterward by yourself, or even record the conversation. This isn't ridiculous. It's important.

To help get you started on those thought processes and conversations, here are some examples:

Your sense of humor lights up a room. You are a social butterfly. You are really shy, and it's very sweet. Once people can get you to open up, you're a fountain of good jokes, insights, and love. You are complicated. You have long hair that whips around in the wind and makes you look like a Greek goddess. You have the pride of a lioness. You are a diligent worker. You inspire other people. You are honest. You get all the questions right on *Jeopardy*. You get none of the questions right on *Jeopardy*. Your laugh brings joy to everyone around you. You are ambitious and excellent at your job. You are a good mother. You are a good grandmother. You take care of people in a very real way. You are an excellent listener. You give great hugs. You have dreams, and you are going places. You make a positive impact just by existing, and for that you should be proud.

There are millions of things about you that are worthy of love, and they all come together in a brilliant mosaic. Meditate on them. Own them. Love them. They are who you are, and you are worthy of every single one of these beautiful qualities. You are worthy of every drop of affirmation you have ever received. You deserve love for millions of reasons. Now it is time to accept the love that the people in your life are throwing your way and to permit yourself to bask in it.

Loving your existential self

As important as our physical and non-physical selves are, the final kind of self-love may be the most powerful. This self-love is the self-love of nature—the self-love that has been a part of you since you were in your mother's womb. It says that you are worthy by the simple fact of your existence. This self-love is not predicated on how you look, how you act, how you think, or how you feel. It is permanent and unconditional.

Existential self-love says that you are worthy *no matter what.* It says that love isn't based on characteristics. It demands that you love yourself and all other beings unconditionally, with profoundly open arms. No matter what you have done in your past, what you may do in your future, and what things may befall you in between, you are an integral part of the complex web of life, and therefore you are worthy of loveliness and composed of beauty. The world would not be the same without you. You are necessary and important.

Your inherent worth is not predicated on social status, on being funny or smart, or on living up to anyone's expectations, your own or otherwise. It is not predicated on success or failure. It is not predicated on your personality. It is not predicated on what you choose to do with your life or how much you earn. It is inherent in you as a woman, as a part of the universe, as a being with feelings, a heart, and a place in the cosmos. You are worthy of love by the simple fact of your existence. You may not be good at loving yourself right now. Other people may wax and wane with regard to how well they love you. But you are unavoidably worthy of love *all the time,* at home in the love of the world. It doesn't always feel that way, no. But it is there, and you deserve it.

Existential self-love undergirds all the other kinds of self-love. It is the bedrock of acceptance, forgiveness, patience, and every other practice I urge you to develop in your relationship with yourself. It is the most important tool for your healing. Why? You must be forgiven for forgiveness to work its magic. You must accept what has happened to you and who you are. You must have patience for yourself as you move beyond who you are and into a brighter future. Existential self-love assures that those things can happen.

Other kinds of love come and go. If you depend on them and they falter for any reason, your relationship with yourself can be hurt. Existential self-love, however, puts its foot down. It says no to anything that attempts to judge you or rob you of self-esteem. It sets a firm foundation for all the self-loving behaviors you live out in your life. Personally, I never would have triumphed over my acne and begun to go out in public if I didn't believe so firmly in my rightness as a human being removed from judgment. Six million thumbs up for existential self-love and for all the brilliant, transformative ways in which it works in women's lives.

Self-love tips

○ **Lavish love on specific characteristics.**

Heaping love on yourself can be so much fun and can make you excited to be you. Just be careful not to become overly attached to impermanent traits.

○ **Make a list of things to love about yourself.**

Inventory your own mind, and dig around in the minds of others. When I am struggling to believe something about myself, I go looking for evidence. I ask my mother: "I really am good at this sort of thing, aren't I?" "Yes!" she always says. And I believe her, especially when she provides specific examples of my successes. Specificity in this kind of love is quite important. We need concrete examples to hang our hats on.

Make this list visible. Tape it up where you'll see it daily, maybe several times a day. Or commit to adding one thing to the list every day. Before you know it, you'll have hundreds of positive qualities to celebrate. The more you remind yourself of what's exciting and lovable about you, the more excited you will be to be in your own skin.

○ **Cover up the mirror.**

One experiment I like to recommend is forgoing looking in the mirror. It works best if you can avoid mirrors entirely, though it's understandable if you have to look quickly to make sure your buttons aren't crooked before you rush out the door.

Before beginning this experiment, allot a specific amount of time for it. A month would be great; a week might be plenty; one day would be a good start. Do your best to commit to that time period. The longer you go without looking in the mirror, the greater your results will probably be.

One fact of human nature is that we tend to focus on our flaws. When I constantly encountered mirrors, I obsessed over the flaws. I had learned them so well that I could hardly see anything else. Shutting off my ability to use a mirror cut off that nitpicking. It also prevented my face from seeming so ho-hum. Being exposed to my face so many times a day made it seem boring and ordinary, rarely beautiful, and never exotic.

Once, I lived in the wilderness without mirrors for several weeks. When I returned to civilization, I did not recognize myself. Who's that woman with the beautiful golden locks? Who's the lady with the radiant skin, full lips, and lovely figure? I hadn't seen myself in weeks, and I had forgotten what I looked like. Upon my return, I regarded myself with the eyes of an objective observer for the first time. I was not just ordinary. I was beautiful. I was even exotic.

Of course, thinking yourself beautiful is not the same as loving yourself. In fact, the beauty effect is just one positive effect of covering the mirror. The other is simple, but arguably more important: covering the mirror lessens the importance of image in your relationship with yourself. It was amazing for me to learn how much of my negativity came from my looks, and how much of my mental wellness had to do with self-consciousness about my appearance. Try covering your mirrors, or at least looking in them less often, and experience the removal of a world of concern and self-doubt.

○ **Think about the way you treat people you love, and then treat yourself that way.**

Consider your friends, mother, sister, daughter, or other women in your life. How deserving of love are they? How well do you treat them? Do you accept them, forgive them, have patience for them? Do you embrace and cherish them, coaching and nourishing rather than castigating and doubting?

Just about every woman I have ever met treats herself more harshly than she does others. Why? Fear and habit, I think. We fear rejection, so we set high expectations for ourselves, and we cultivate these habits over time so much that we don't even notice that we are doing so. But we are. Daily.

How much love do you wish your friends and family members felt for themselves? How badly do you wish that they would realize how lovely and good they are? How much do you want everyone in your life to experience profound wellness, peace, and self-esteem? How radically worthy do you find so many people who doubt and question themselves?

All of us are engaged in this game. We give other people so much leeway. It is time to extend that flexibility to yourself. If other people are worthy of love no matter how human and flawed they are, then you are, too.

○ **Consider spiritual practices that enrich your sense of inherent self-worth.**

Many people find it helpful to locate love in the cosmos by thinking that God or the universe is love. If you are among them, focus on that source of love. Make it central to your life. Cultivate a spiritual life and spiritual practices that orient you around it. You are inherently worthy as a part of the cosmos, however you might see it. It is up to you to allow yourself to feel that worth.

"The winds of grace are always blowing," someone once said to me. "All you have to do is lift your sails."

○ **Consider therapy.**

I have two therapists. I do not believe this indicates that there is something "wrong" with me. Actually, I think the fact that I seek therapy means that there is something "right" with me. It means that I am taking specific steps to become a better and happier human being.

We all have baggage. We all have histories. And complex things happen to us day in and day out. Therapy is one of many tools that can help. If you struggle to love yourself, working through your past and your obstacles to self-love with a therapist is a very real and effective way to overcome it all.

○ **Deconstruct negative thoughts about yourself.**

Learning where negative thoughts come from is one of the most powerful things you can do for your ability to love yourself. Just as you have to accept what has made you who you are today, you also have to understand those things and where they have come from in order to let them go. If you don't understand what's in the way of your self-love, how can you ever get around it? That's like going into battle without knowing where the enemy troops are. The better you know what the troops are up to, the better your chance of overcoming those obstacles. Only with real introspection, reconciliation, and work can you learn what's keeping you down. Then, after tearing it down, you have (mostly) fresh ground on which to build self-love in its place.

○ **Accept what you cannot control.**

On and off throughout my life I stumble upon the same quote, and every time I find it useful: "Grant me the grace to accept the things I cannot change, the courage to change the things I can, and the wisdom to know the difference." To which I can only say, "Amen." So many things in this world are out of our control. The set of genes you have is one of them. What has happened to you in your life so far is another. How other people think and behave also go on that list. What can you do about it all? Nothing.

You have the power to choose your *reactions* to these things. You can choose to be kept down, or you can rise up and chart your own path forward. But you can't change those things that are out of your control. Acceptance is the only way.

Accepting the things you cannot change liberates you from unrealistic expectations, enables you to make peace with your body and your life, and frees you to embrace the future. For example, I cannot change the fact that I have PCOS, which makes it hard for my metabolism to work properly sometimes. But I can change my habits. I can reduce my stress. I can keep my diet as clean as possible. And I do. It frees me from feeling like beating myself up when the cysts rear their ugly heads. I cannot punish myself if I accept that the problem is out of my control. All I can do is let go and move forward.

○ **Cultivate patience for your progress.**

Just as it is important to accept what you cannot control, you must forgive the things you perceive as being within your control. Progress takes time. You will never do anything perfectly immediately, including developing a healthier body or a positive relationship with yourself. This has been one of the hardest points for me to navigate in my own health journey.

I firmly believe that everything that happens in the body is a response to a specific cause. For example, I always believed that my acne was caused by something I was doing or eating. But I could not figure it out what it was. For three years, I hated my acne with unparalleled fury. I thought that I should have been able to control it, but I couldn't.

Over time, I learned about the specifics of my body chemistry, which led me to some solutions. More importantly, however, I learned how crucial it was to forgive myself for being unable to heal the acne right away. There was no way I could do it in a day, a week, a month, or even a year. I could only continue to do my best and to forgive myself as I kept trying new things and learning. It took a very long time. There was a lot to learn. But accepting that the road would be bumpy and forgiving myself along the way made the journey infinitely more pleasant.

* * *

These are powerful tips that I have used myself and have witnessed others benefit greatly from. Therapy may be the most important of all. I can't know what specific skeletons are in your closet, and I can't speak directly to you about your unique blocks to self-love. You have to wrestle with those specifics on your own, or in the company of good friends and good doctors.

Because I can't speak to your own skeletons, I must close this section with a simple call to pay attention to self-love. Know that you are worthy of it, and that if you struggle for it, many tools are available to you. As you move forward, let acceptance, forgiveness, patience, spiritual practices, and daily reminders of your self-worth as a physical, non-physical, and existential being support you. These tools have given me the ability to love myself and to stand by myself in the face of enormous forces urging me to do otherwise. They also, delightfully, formed the bedrock of my ability to be a relentlessly and unapologetically sexy woman. It is yours for the taking, now, to do the same.

Self-Determined Sex Appeal

Just about everyone who is sexy and knows it is in on a secret. I have hinted at it multiple times, but I have yet to state it outright. You are ready now. The secret is this:

**You are the one who determines
how sexy you are.**

It is not your boyfriend. It is not your friends. It is not the crowd of people in the supermarket. Sure, they judge you. They are human beings—they can't help it. But their judgment has nothing to do with how you feel about and relate to yourself. Moreover, the woman they see is predicated on what you present to them. Sex appeal lives in the space between you and the people around you. But it starts with you. It *has* to.

"Sexy" is a funny concept. To be honest, I wake up every morning dazed by the reality that I have written a book on the subject. When I tell my feminist friends about it (to be clear: all my friends are feminists), they gasp in horror. "Are you for real, woman?" Yes, I am. "Do you realize that you are promoting womanhood based on appearances? Aren't you encouraging women to become sex objects even more than they were before? Don't you feel guilty about that?" Er, no. That's not what I'm doing. At least that is not my intention.

Does this book promote womanhood based on appearances? Somewhat. It acknowledges that appearances are important. You can't escape them. But this book does not promote an empty shell of womanhood that relies on meeting appearance-based norms. Explicitly, it does *not*. *I do not*. As I've said, sex appeal *starts with you* and your health. Sexiness lives in your heart and in your bones. It is threaded throughout every fiber of your natural being. The only thing you have to do to be sexy is to feel it, believe it, and embody it.

* * *

One of the most revelatory experiences I have ever had was in my early days as a writer and a blogger. I had blogged for quite some time but had only recently made the jump to a more ambitious kind of blogging. I redesigned my website. I overhauled my methods and crafted more robust blog posts. I started consulting women officially on diet and body image issues. I self-published materials on overcoming certain health conditions. To be successful in those endeavors, however, I had to find answers to the questions: "How do I get people to trust me? Why should they trust me? Who am I to be giving this kind of advice?"

It turns out that no one treated me like a professional until I started acting like one. No one slapped a blue ribbon on me and told me I had made it. The same goes for any characteristic or person you want to be, *especially* sexy. No one is going to do that work for you. No one is going to change who you are or how you feel about your life. Who you are is in your hands. How sexy you are is within your power. You just have to own it and stride defiantly onward.

The secret to sex appeal is that *you* determine how sexy you are. Don't let the idea scare you off—not this far along in the process. It is based on several simple steps, which I detail and help you implement below. It relies on principles I have already covered. First and foremost, it relies on self-love. In line with self-love, sexiness requires that you be allied with and accepting of your body. It requires that you be on its side, and proudly so. This enables you to define your own notion of what it means to be and to feel sexy. As you do so, you will become more and more excited to be in the skin you are in.

Choosing and feeling sexy
makes you appear sexy

Much as I stand by the idea that sexiness is an internal feeling, that doesn't stop me or you from being human. We want to be liked. We want to be attractive. We want to feel sexy, and we want other people to recognize it.

Being seen as sexy follows naturally from demonstrating that you feel sexy. When you decide to be sexy, others listen. Just as I made the choice to be a professional, I also chose to own my sexiness. I chose to be a sexy woman. And now I am. Think of the sexy people in your life. Think of sexy things that people do. Imagine a person who unashamedly wears flattering clothes, walks with his chin up, smiles at people he passes on the street, and sits and moves like he owns and is comfortable in his body even if he is unattractive. Compare him to someone with a perfect body who slumps his shoulders, picks at the sleeve of his sweater, and feels self-conscious about it all. Who would you rather date? Confidence is key. Fearlessness is key. Self-determination is key.

* * *

Making the decision to be sexy enables other people to think that you are sexy. Of course they might do so on their own, but they are helped enormously by your decision. If you are convinced that you are a sexy woman, other people will find it much easier to believe you.

Choosing to be sexy changes the way you walk and the way you talk, and many other things besides. It makes it easier to smile. It makes it easier to laugh. It makes it easier to *strut*—to walk down the street with confidence, pride, and allegiance to your natural body. Choosing sexiness presents you to the world as a sexy human being, and this is precisely how the gap is bridged between you and the rest of the world.

A too-brief note regarding inclusivity

This book has the potential to be read only gender normatively and heterosexually. I speak broadly about feminine norms that may not apply to homosexual, queer, transgendered, or other non-traditionally oriented people. I acknowledge that fact openly. This just so happens to be a book directed at people who identify as female and/or as women because there are specific problems that plague this demographic in and of itself.

Nonetheless, I remain firm in my conviction that any and all people can suffer from the problems I deal with in this book, whether heterosexual, homosexual, queer, male, female, or anything else, and all are welcome to read and participate in it.

To that end, I have done my best to maintain a focus on women's issues and the womanly community while still using inclusive language. Moreover, several times in the book I mention the community of beauty and competition between women. This idea does not apply only to competition between women for men's attention, but also to acknowledgement and beauty in general, social problems that exist in and among all of us. The community of beauty is among women, but it is also, importantly, among all human beings.

Sexy tips

Now that we've talked the talk, it's time to walk the walk. You probably won't roll over tomorrow morning and think, "I believe I am worthy of sex appeal for the first time in my life!" This would be nice, but chances are it won't happen without digging deep into your thoughts and habits and changing them over time. This is where my sexy tips come into play. Learn and practice them until they become second nature.

○ **Accept, forgive, and love yourself.**

Acceptance is the cornerstone of sex appeal, just as it is the cornerstone of self-love and health. Accepting yourself is the number one thing you must do before you start on any part of the *Sexy by Nature* journey. Period.

I never loved my body until I got on its side and said, "I understand." Try putting yourself in the "shoes" of your body. How might your body tell the story of your life and health? Might it say, "I'm trying as hard as I can, but drugs, unhealthy foods, and stress have been keeping me down"? Chances are quite good that it would. Your body is not evil. It's not stupid. It's not out to get you. It is doing its best to heal and to be sexy. It has just faced significant obstacles along the way.

Accepting your body as it is today enables you to forgive past transgressions and move into the future with forgiveness. You have been hurt, but working together with your body fosters healing. Acceptance gives you a means by which to sign a peace treaty and feel at home in your body. Acceptance gives you a comfortable base off of which you can build excitement. Acceptance gives you the power to stand up for your body and flip the bird to anyone and anything telling you to do otherwise. The more you accept your body and move forward *together* toward a healthier, sexier you, the more pride and passion you can have for your body. Acceptance will forever be the anchor of your self-worth and sexiness.

○ **Be yourself.**

There is no reason to adopt behaviors or looks that are not you. You are your sexiest self when you are yourself. If you try to be someone you are not, you won't be the only one who feels weird; other people will feel weird, too. Humans have a strong sense for discomfort and dishonesty. If you try to be someone else, it will show. Don't let society mold you into someone you are not. Trying to be someone else would be playing by the worst of the old rules—not a good idea.

> You are your sexiest self when you are yourself.

Being yourself is probably the most powerful force for sex appeal in the whole book. Here's a quick example from my own life. I go out dancing several nights a week. One of the most important lessons I have learned in doing so is that I should never wear clothing that doesn't feel "me." Sometimes I pick out fashionable, sexy outfits that look great on me in dressing room mirrors—a slinky red dress, for example. But when I wear these things, I feel...not me. I don't dance as well. I don't hold my chin up. I don't make eye contact and wink. That happens only when I wear a beat-up pair of jeans. I might not look like a stereotypical salsa dancer, but I look like me. And is there ever a difference in the way I dance! Because I feel comfortable, unapologetic, and sexy as myself, the nights when I wear my usual clothes are my best nights of dancing. I have more fun. Men approach me more. I get more compliments on my dancing—and on the way I live my life. People are drawn to it. Being comfortable in your own skin is the best thing you can do to announce to the world that you are sexy and that everyone had damn well better pay attention (should you want them to).

○ **Eat right.**

Feeding your body good foods is unimaginably important for sex appeal, and for a long list of reasons. For one, the healthier you are, the better support your body has for mental health. Without a healthy brain, it's almost impossible to be happy, be at peace, be confident, or live well. The healthier you are, the easier it is to feel positive emotion.

You'll also have better energy and less pain if you eat well—two things that can boost your excitement to be in the skin you're in. The more healing you do and the more pain you eliminate, the more you can love and trust your body. Healing demonstrates that treating your body well *works;* the more love you heap on your body, the more it loves you back. The more you take care of yourself, the more you are rewarded with positive health and energy.

Finally, the more healing you do, the more physically attractive you can feel and become. As you heal, you will lose weight if you need to. Your skin will clear. Your hair will become shinier. Your muscles will firm up. You will tan more easily and burn much less often. Your teeth can even whiten and fill in their own cavities. The more healing you do, the sexier you become.

○ Dance. (Or move.)

I may be a bit biased on this score, but I think you should dance. Dance frequently, dance freely, dance joyfully, dance peacefully, dance wildly. Dance whatever you are feeling, whatever moves you and your body in the moment. The reason I love dancing so much is that it facilitates for me exactly what I am trying to do with this book: It puts me in my own body. It makes me feel at home. It makes me feel free, playful, and alive. It's not about dancing in an alluring fashion—though that *is* nice. It is, instead, about bodily movement. It's about power. It's about joy.

I recommend dancing in your kitchen first and foremost—as often as you can. A fun thing to do is to challenge yourself to dance to one song every day for a month. Some women in my blogging community tried that last year and loved it. Moving feels good. And moving with the freedom just to *be* in your body and connect with your body helps turn you into a woman who is excited and grateful to have such a powerful body.

If you don't like dancing, no matter. Try another kind of movement. Get into the flow of your body. Harmonize with it. Become one with your strongly muscled legs as you cycle over a mountain pass. Feel your heart beat in yoga class. Run in time with your lungs and your breath as you power up steps and over bridges. Find a movement that makes you come alive, and go out and do it. What your sex appeal needs is for your body to come alive.

○ Develop skills and passions.

The better you are at things, the more you love who you are and are proud of yourself. These can be physical endeavors that give you faith in your physical body, or they can be solely mental endeavors. It doesn't matter. The basic premise is that skills and passions are sexy. Certain passions can be so strong that they override all the other tricks for sexiness that I talk about in this book, making you excited and sexy all on their own.

Examples abound. My love interests have almost always been musicians. Listening to them play so passionately, watching them display their talents onstage—these things make musicians appealing to me. If this level of radiant excellence isn't sexy, I don't know what is.

In my own life, I could point to passions like dance that make me feel sexy. But dance feels a bit like cheating because dance and other physical endeavors are commonly regarded as sexy passions. A more powerful example is my work as an aspiring philosopher. I spend the vast majority of my time in the library reading books by thinkers like Plato, Kant, Nietzsche, and Heidegger. I wear thick glasses. The ninety-five books I have borrowed from the library comprise several towers on my bedroom floor. This, I think, is one of the sexiest things about me—maybe even the most. It's a passion that makes me love who I am in a profound way. It makes me feel powerful and worthy and proud. These kinds of endeavors can do the same for you.

Developing skills and passions unrelated to your physicality might be especially useful if you have a great deal of psychological and physiological healing ahead of you. If developing a positive relationship with your body will be a long journey for you, rely more on tools that can empower you outside of physicality. You can have skills that make you sexy no matter where in your health journey you are. Sexiness is not just about how you look. It's about who you are, and about accepting and loving your whole self.

○ **Practice gratitude for your body.**

Your body is a powerful thing. Even if you deal with significant health issues or disabilities, the things that are right with your body still vastly outnumber the things that are wrong. Your heart beats. Your lungs breathe. Your muscles propel movement. You can see, hear, smell, taste, and touch. Even better, you can gaze, listen, savor, delight, and feel. You can dance. You can sing. You can relax and laugh and experience emotions and make love and live, all because your body provides you with the foundation to do so.

Your body is a part of the intricate billion-year-long saga of life on this planet. What an amazing thing to be a part of! And for this thing to give you so much life and experience! Admittedly, it isn't all roses. It isn't all smiles. But it is *life,* and your body gives you the ability and the honor to live it.

Praying or meditating daily can be a great way to practice gratitude and awe for your body. Writing down reminders and taping them to your wall, your desk, your steering wheel, or your mirror can also work wonders. One thing I liked to do in my college years was to write important quotes and points of gratitude on a few pairs of pants so that they were always with me. I got funny stares sometimes, but more often than not people loved the idea. Even if they didn't, it didn't matter a lick to me. You might also try wearing jewelry that reminds you of certain things. Anything you do to enhance the gratitude you feel for your life and your body will make you a happier person. Psychological studies have proven this a million times over.

Showing gratitude for your body will help you treat yourself better, too. This has been demonstrated by the lives of so many women who have overcome body image issues. Your body is a miracle. Don't let anyone convince you otherwise.

○ **Turn off the sexy switch.**

Even though I consider myself a sexy person, I do not need to be dressed up all the time. In fact, I'm currently in a library with unwashed hair, no makeup, and an outfit I am not particularly fond of. I can still smile confidently at the people around me (this would have been impossible for me years ago) because my self-worth is more than my physicality. I am far more than just a sexual human being. You are far more than just a sexual human being. You are delightful, powerful, intelligent, witty, and fun. You do not need to present yourself as sexy all the time.

Turning off the need to be attractive and just letting yourself be is one of the most powerful things you can do for your sex appeal. It may seem counterintuitive, but it's true. Why? Because it reminds you that you are more than appearances. Your worth is inherent. You do not need other people to be sexy. You do not need mascara, or lipstick, or sheer tops or short-shorts or high heels. You *are* sexy by your very nature. The more you believe that, the more you can live it, and the more you are enabled to feel and be sexy in the totality of your life.

When your sexy feelings are internal and you believe in your basic worth as a desirable human being, you don't need to look or be perfect. On some days you might present yourself "better" or differently, and on other days you might choose to wear sweatpants. That's okay. No one can rob you of your sexuality. You are sexy whenever you choose to be.

○ **Spend time in nature or alone.**

There are few better ways to remind yourself of the naturalness of your body than to get out into the natural world. This may seem like a stretch—will it really make you feel sexy?—but it cultivates your relationship with yourself and your appreciation for the glory of your natural body. What's more, stepping out of the rat race and into a calm world on your own re-centers you. Much as I love and am married to the principles I espouse in this book, it's easy for the world to reach out and trip me up from time to time. Getting out into the woods or onto a mountaintop helps me feel whole and natural again and gives me the refreshing dose of beauty and peace that I need to return to city life with my chin held high.

If nature's not for you, consider retreating to a spa or a safe space such as a family member's home. Vacations are good for you. Done right, they can enhance your feelings of peace and self-worth.

○ **Fake it 'til you make it.**

How do you feel sexy? How do you act sexy? Aside from having all the right ideas in place in your head, you leap into it. You just start. If it's new to you, that's okay. Give it a go and learn over time. You might be amazed at what happens!

What does sexy look like? I can't tell you for certain because it is different for every woman. What do you imagine sexy people do? Here are some ideas—I have done these things often:

○ Put on a big smile.

○ Wear your favorite skirt.

○ Strut down the street. Practice doing it with no one around first if that's easier.

○ Listen to sexy pump-up music.

○ Sway your hips as you walk around getting ready in the morning.

○ Wear new lingerie under your work clothes.

○ Do a sexy dance while you cook your meals.

○ Make sure that whatever you wear is flattering.

○ Wear your favorite color as often as possible.

○ Smile at the strangers you pass.

○ Pull your shoulders back and tip your head up.

○ Buy yourself a flower on the way to work.

Give these things a try even if you don't feel it. Even if it feels alien, wrong, or silly. Trust me, there are a lot of silly ideas rooted deep in your heart trying to keep you from the glory of proud sexuality. Say no, give sexy practices a go, and see what happens. Put on the sexy mantle.

Fake it, and all of a sudden you'll find that you've made it.

○ **Care for yourself like a worthy and sexy being.**

Just as I learned that I had to treat myself like a professional before anyone else would treat me like one, I must treat myself like I am sexy. What does this mean? I take luxurious baths from time to time because I deserve them. I set aside time to moisturize my skin. I wear clothing that flatters me. I do stretches and yoga. I occasionally take the time to pamper myself in ways that extend beyond diet and exercise, which makes me feel and be sexier and deepens my level of intimacy with my body.

The more sexy attention you give yourself, the more worthy of this kind of attention you will feel. Moreover, your pride in and allegiance to your sexual worth will skyrocket. Treating yourself like a sexy human being sets a standard that you should never lower. All the people in your life, especially those with whom you share a romantic connection, need to live up to this standard. You are worthy of sexiness. You are worthy of appreciation, love, and desire. Give it to yourself. Your actions are the ones that matter most.

Fearlessness

One hot summer night, long after sunset, I was sitting on the bank of the Charles River with one of my wisest friends. The river drifted amiably by. Bats swooped in and out. The moon was shining. It was a quiet moment—an uncommon thing in Boston. My friend, sitting cross-legged next to me on the grass, said something that changed my life. He said, "Stef, everything I do in life is an act of fear or an act of love." He went on to tell me that his goal in life was to eliminate fear and to do everything out of love. We talked for a while longer on the topic, but my world had already shifted. He was right. Fear lives on one bank, and love on the other.

What does this have to do with *Sexy by Nature*? Just about everything. Fear is what drives us to be hard on ourselves. Fear makes us scared of judgment. Fear makes us look the other way when we pass strangers on the sidewalk. Fear is an inherently human thing, a part of our nature. My quest as an empowered and natural woman, however, is to stop being so afraid of everything. I cannot fear rejection. I cannot fear judgment. I cannot live my life hidden in the shadows, too afraid of losing love to be open enough to give or receive it. This final section of the book is about confidence. It's about strutting. It's about sex appeal. It's about being hot and feeling hot and owning it. For the sake of our bodies and selves, it is imperative that this book close on fearlessness.

> Strutting is an act of fearless self-love.

Strutting is an act of fearless self-love. Every time I step out the door and raise my chin, it's an act of fierce allegiance to self-worth, to self-love, and to being myself despite everything that tells me to do otherwise. Fearlessly being myself is the most natural thing I can do. As such, it's one of the most physically and mentally healthy things I can do. I embrace my story. I embrace my body and my spirit and all of who I am. And I step out into the world with so much pride and love that no amount of external pressure is going to tear me down.

The community of beauty

I have never understood and will never understand the idea that beauty is relative. When I used to come across beautiful women, my first instinct was to feel jealous or resentful. It almost felt as though her beauty made it less possible for me to be beautiful, too. She was stealing *my* spotlight, *my* beauty.

This idea—which lives in the hearts of all of us, I think—makes it seem as though there's a limited amount of beauty in the world, and not everybody can have it. To this I say *no way!* Seriously, ladies. Why did I ever think that another woman's beauty lessened my own? Why did it threaten me? Another woman's beauty might cause some people to find her more attractive than I am, but there are billions of men and women in the world, and there's a decent chance that some people might find *me* more attractive.

Or perhaps this woman achieves some ideal of beauty that no woman could ever match. Fine. But the big question of who she is and what other qualities she possesses rises up in response. Does her physical appearance have anything to do with who she really is? Perhaps she is physically striking, but don't we all have deeper beauty? Isn't it mostly what's on the inside that counts?

More important than all else, however, we must ask ourselves: Why compare at all? Why compete?

Just because one woman is beautiful does not mean that you are *less*. There is no absolute amount of beauty in the world that is doled out unequally among women. There is zero reason to resent her. Why not be happy for her instead? Why not be excited by how much beauty the world has to offer? Even if a beautiful woman catches more eyes at the bar, it doesn't mean anything for your sex appeal. Your sex appeal is exactly the same as it was when you walked into the bar. And it is predicated on your story and your life and your confidence and nothing else.

We are all beautiful. Better, we can all feel beautiful, and we can acknowledge each other's beauty. We don't need to be threatened by each other. In fact, we would do well to work together rather than against each other. There's way too much negativity in the world to let ourselves do that to each other anymore. What business do we have multiplying that negativity and making it even harder to feel and be beautiful?

We are all *different*. We are all *unique*. This is true of women's personalities as well as women's physical bodies. We exist in a *community of beauty*. We are in this together. We all deal with insecurities. We all feel pain. We all worry about what others think of us. Instead of living in fear and trying to tear each other down, wouldn't we be better served by supporting each other? We have the power to share love and beauty, so let's throw fear out the window and roar together.

Steps to fearlessness

Just as I have shared the means by which I have enhanced my feelings of self-love and sexiness, I have also explored the world of courage as it relates to beauty. Below are the seven steps that I and thousands of women in my community have relied on that have the power to transform you into a fearlessly embodied woman.

Step 1: Love yourself unconditionally

Love is the most important of all the steps, the same as it is for feeling sexy. How do you overcome a fear of rejection? Build up so much love in your life that rejection becomes meaningless. You cannot be upset with yourself for things you cannot change. I cannot hate my imperfect ovaries. I cannot hate my acne. I cannot hate my body for not being perfect. I can only love it for doing its best. I embrace it for everything it has been, everything it is, and everything it is going to be. I even forgive myself for starving myself in the past. I have to—there is no other option. My eyes are on the future, and my love, acceptance, and forgiveness for myself are my top priorities as I move forward.

So what does it matter if a stranger likes you or not, or is attracted to you or not? Does this person's opinion of you say anything about who you are? The same goes for the people who are close to you. If they do not like or love you for who you are, what are they doing in your life? Life is too short to spend it around people who make you feel bad about yourself. I am not telling you that you must break up with friends or acquaintances. I am, however, urging you to consider the role they play in your life. When self-love is the bedrock of health and happiness, it's important to prioritize it as highly as you can.

Step 2: Develop pride

Love might be enough to get you most of the way there, but in my experience, there's so much negativity and potential for rejection and hurt out there that love has to be bolstered by unapologetic pride. You could say that the best defense is a strong offense.

In saying "offense," I am not advocating that you attack the people around you. Rather, project your self-love and self-worth out into the world. Put it out there before anyone has a chance to say no. This way, your love is already standing at attention whenever potential pain comes your way. Be proud of who you are. Be proud of your story and your body and everything you are and do. Stand by your body and your identity first and foremost. Anything that comes up against them should be immediately discarded.

Discarding painful events is not the easiest thing to do, especially when someone in whom you are invested rejects you. Sometimes friends and romantic interests don't call back. It happens to all of us. Do not doubt yourself in the face of rejection. In the end, you cannot control anyone's thoughts but your own. If you don't like me, that's fine. I love myself. I know I am worthy despite anything that's thrown my way.

Pride is not arrogance. It does not mean thinking that you are better than anyone else. It means being human and messing up and needing forgiveness and having it all be okay anyway. You are always good enough. You are yourself, and you deserve your own loyalty. You have no option to be anyone or anything else. So own it. Be proud of being a natural woman. Stand up for empowered womanhood. Be excited to be a woman who says yes to confidence and no to fear. You and your body have nothing to apologize for. You are unapologetically who you are, and no one can take that away from you.

Step 3: Acknowledge other people's contexts

When I go out to a bar or a club and try to make friends, not everyone is receptive. Plenty of people aren't interested. They might already have a significant other or plenty of friends. Or they just might not feel a spark with me and my particular personality. Fine. Seriously, it's okay! It's not always easy, but we have to let these things go. One of the best ways to do so is to remember that each person has his or her own story and context. You might feel rejected, but what if the people you are trying to engage are under a significant amount of stress, are themselves self-conscious, or are preoccupied with something? You never know what's going on inside another person's head. People cannot be faulted for having their own feelings and doing their best to get through each day. Acknowledge that any rejection you feel is probably not meant to hurt you, and move forward feeling better for that fact.

Step 4: Don't chase affirmation

As obvious as this step might seem, it's an easy one to forget. As I began to build confidence and noticed that people were actually quite receptive to my confident winks, I started to garner positive attention. It was great! Positive attention and happy interactions are the stuff that living is *for*. On the other hand, on occasion I forget my lessons about internal love and self-worth and get wrapped up in tallying appreciative nods.

The trick is to step back and think of the big picture. As lovely as it is to be confident, feel sexy, and develop flirtatious and positive interactions with other people, affirmation cannot be the ultimate goal. Affirmation from the outside is secondary to the love and worth you have built up on the inside. You are *always* lovable, sexy, and worthy. You are so many powerful and lovely things as a natural woman. When others like these things, you have the opportunity to interact based on them. But interaction cannot be your sole goal. When it is, self-consciousness tends to rear its ugly head. Negative thoughts leak in. Doubt and judgment leak in. That's bad news. Shut it off. Remember the good stuff. Worth is inherent. Love is unconditional. *These* are the foundations of radiant womanhood.

Step 5: Be kind first

On the banks of the Charles River, my friend enlightened me to the power that fear has over our lives. The more I thought about it, the more I understood what he was getting at. The more I integrated this idea in my life, the more my outgoing, happy behavior took on a serious, world-changing overtone.

As much as we live in fear, so do all the people around us. If you look away because you are afraid of rejection, then the person across from you who looks away is doing the same thing. Everyone wants love, and everyone fears rejection. Interactions between people get cut off from both sides. If you are standing on one end of a football field and a potential friend is standing on the other, what happens if you both send out only 20 yards worth of openness and kindness? You never meet, that's what. There's still 60 yards of open grass between you. The kindness quota is not met, and because of fear, you both miss out on friendship.

It takes immense courage, but if you want to have positive interactions with strangers, sometimes you have to give it up first. I give it the full 100 yards. Smiling, looking unafraid, saying hello...

these are all ways to show other people that I am kind. They make all the difference. If I approached people with defensiveness and fear, they'd have little reason to trust me or to be interested in me. Approaching others with openness—even giving them compliments, asking how they are doing, or winking—is one of the best way to lower walls.

A lot of women miss out on opportunities to flirt, I think, because their prospects are just as afraid. Sometimes I wonder if we all walk around with no one to talk to only because we haven't started talking first. The same goes for flirting, romancing, and the like.

Everyone is afraid. Be the first person to be step up, smile, and open up. Be the first person to create a connection and assure a safe space for interaction. These are the actions of which real loving womanhood, sexy empowerment, and positive change in the world are made.

Step 6: Practice eye contact

One of the best ways to gain confidence is to practice making eye contact. The more I do it, the more I learn how many positive effects it has on me and the world. This knowledge makes me all the more eager to interact and all the more excited about going out and being myself.

Begin practicing with people you are not attracted to and whom you know already love you—friends, colleagues, your mother. Push through awkward moments. The awkward moments will happen, but experiencing them can teach you that there is nothing to fear beyond them. Experiencing the awkwardness and realizing how unimportant it is melted my discomfort. There is nothing earth-shattering about a bit of eye contact. Just you and another person. The awkwardness fades and the delight roars in.

After familiar faces, graduate to strangers. I did this with a mantra running through my head: "I have nothing to lose, I have nothing to lose." If they did not respond positively to me, that was fine. They just might have been having a bad day. Yet despite knowing this, I was constantly rewarded. People almost always smiled back. Trust me when I tell you that if you open up to strangers in this small way, you will be delighted by positive responses a million times more often than you will be ignored, rejected, or hurt.

The final challenge is to begin making eye contact with people you find attractive (whether or not you are currently pursuing romance). I have been working on this one for years, and I still catch myself being bashful more than I'd like to. Nonetheless, you have nothing to lose. Don't go into the interactions anticipating affirmation. Don't set expectations. Just open up and see what happens. Dare to look people in the eyes. Dare to smile. Dare to be kind. That's all it is, really: openness and kindness and possibility. That practice and the joy that comes from it makes all the fearless difference.

Step 7: Leap

In this final step, there is nothing left to do but *leap*.

On page 297, I share a story about professionalism. At the beginning of my career, I learned very quickly that no one was going to treat me like a professional unless I was one. Eventually I became a fairly successful professional woman. This never would have happened if I hadn't put on my big-girl shoes and stepped into that role on my own.

The same thing goes for sexiness, as well as just about any other characteristic you might desire to have. I didn't become sexy until I decided to be sexy. I didn't feel sexy until I decided to allow myself to do so. I didn't come across as sexy until I let my real self shine. I never would have been able to do any of these things if I didn't have the courage to leap into radical self-love and pride.

The key is to love yourself so fiercely and to be so proud of who you are that you have nothing to fear. Then you can just walk out the door and smile. You can be happy and free. Don't carry the weight of self-loathing on your shoulders. Don't fear rejection. Don't worry about what people will think. Instead, wrap yourself in your own love and proud allegiance to your natural body.

This should be as true on "bad" days as it is on "good" days. Trust me when I say that I do have bad ones. Proud and strong as I aspire to be, a very significant part of me is still a little girl in this big, scary world, and I have days when I feel sad, doubt myself, and hate my body. It's okay to have bad days and slip into self-consciousness and fear. Just keep doing your best to make the good ones outnumber the bad. The longer you practice these steps, the more normal it will be for you to forgive yourself, accept and love yourself wholly, and treat yourself with the love and care you deserve.

Something revolutionary

Is all this easier said than done? Perhaps. Though perhaps not. This book has built you up to shed your fear. You have the foods you need to heal yourself. Your relationship with your body is more positive because you are giving it what it needs. You are becoming healthier and more energetic every day. You are overcoming illness and supporting your body. You are learning to love it as it was designed, and you are embracing parts of yourself that are natural and out of your control. You are learning to forgive yourself and to love yourself in the face of great social forces telling you not to. These are extraordinary changes.

Fearless womanhood is perhaps the greatest gift I have ever given myself. It revolutionized my life. I went from sad, hurt, and exhausted to proud, happy in my own skin, and excited to be alive. It took a lot of time, patience, and healing, but the journey has been entirely worth it.

Maybe this idea is silly, but I think the whole thing is a movement. I started calling it that when I had just thirty likes on my Facebook page and one comment on the blog from my mother.

Today, thousands of us are standing up and fearlessly owning our natural bodies. Every day I read new comments about the transformations women are undergoing. Every day I get e-mails about the power these ideas have to revolutionize how women feel about themselves. Every week the movement gains strength: one more woman saying yes to herself and no to norms.

Life in the Western world comes with a lot of amenities, but we are so hard on ourselves and so distanced from our natural bodies that struggle has become the norm. *Sexy by Nature* is about reclaiming the nourishment that brings us happiness and health. It is about values and principles and science and lifestyle. It's about taking ownership of our lives and our health and about revolutionizing womanhood such that we as a community of beautiful, natural women can stand together and proudly love and care for ourselves. This is a movement for health, for love, and for radical empowerment.

In the infancy of my work in my online community, I wrote a tagline for the Facebook page. It still reads this way today:

"Sexy by Nature is a movement. It calls women to own and to love themselves as natural, evolved beings. It demands health, it demands love, and it demands recognition of the power, beauty, and unapologetic radiance of natural womanhood."

Elsewhere it says, "This movement is about empowerment. It's about embracing a woman's body as a natural, evolved organism, and about using whatever experience and knowledge a woman has to nourish and love herself as that organism. Sexy by Nature is about owning womanhood as evolved, as powerful, as individual and real. It's about saying yes to life and no to social norms about body image, identity, presentation, and lifestyle. Most of all, this movement is about being a woman, damn it all, and never, ever apologizing for that fact. This movement is about passion, about community, and about moving forward together in a radical attempt to overthrow American womanhood."

To which I can still say nothing but *amen*.

Epilogue:
On your journey

This book is about a lot of things. When I told people that I wanted to combine a philosophy of natural womanhood with principles of diet, lifestyle, and physical health, just about every person reacted by pretending to take my temperature and asking me if I had walked off the deep end. "You know it's going to be like...600 pages long, right? And no one is going to read it? And it's going to be confusing and complicated and you are just going to make a hot mess of things?"

Yes, I said. Yes, yes, yes, and yes. I knew all those things.

I went ahead and did them anyway.

Physical and psychological wellness are inherently linked; you can't have one without the other. My own experience has demonstrated this to me in a way that makes me more certain of it than of just about every other idea I have ever encountered. Nutrient deficiencies have caused me months of anxiety, insomnia, and panic attacks. Worse, my poor psychological health and negative self-esteem caused me to make restrictive dietary choices that made me infertile, killed my sex drive, and gave me acne. Unfortunately, millions of women wrestle with the same kinds of problems every day.

I could not have written this book without sharing my knowledge and experience of both. They might resonate with you. They might cause a revolution in your own life. They might give you the power you need to take your health, self-confidence, and self-love into your own hands. Goodness, do I ever hope they do.

Regardless of how seriously you take this book and how much you gain from it, I remain firm in my belief that you are worthy of love. You deserve health. You deserve healing. You deserve the kind of energy, positivity, and trust in your body that leads to a life of happiness and wellness. You deserve the real stuff, the stuff that lasts forever, the stuff that makes life worth living. You deserve a sexy body. You deserve to love yourself. You deserve to walk down the street with your head held high. You deserve the gift of your natural body and all the loyalty, love, and affirmation that come with it.

Regardless of the struggles you face in your own journey, you have my love and support and the love and support of the community of women rallied around you. There's an old story that I think is relevant here. A man falls into a hole and can't get out. A preacher walks by, says a prayer for the man, and goes on his way. A librarian walks by and says she'll go get a manual on hole-digging. A construction worker throws the man some tools. But then one of the man's friends sees the man in the hole and leaps down into it. "What are you doing?" the trapped man gasps in response. This isn't good for anybody, he thinks. "Don't worry," the friend replies. "I have been here before, and I know the way out."

The community of women is not one of enemies. It is one of comrades and supporters. The ferocity, joy, and love of the *Sexy by Nature* community prove that to me every day. I have felt so much of your pain, and I hold you in my heart for all the kinds of pain you suffer that are different from and may be much worse than my own. I can't tell you that I have been there exactly, but I have been close, and I believe in you.

Journeys are funny things. They go backward and forward and in circles sometimes. But I tell women in my community that we must always keep our eyes on the future. We might go a step forward and then take 600 steps back, and that's okay. It's about progress. It's about healing. It's about becoming healthier and lovelier and more alive over time. It's about loving ourselves in the process and forgiving whatever pain and hardship bubbles up. You walk forward, you walk around, you walk back. You don't expect perfection. You journey.

You may expect kick-ass results; you have my express permission and even my urging to do so. This book is full of powerful information that will radically overhaul your health, possibly before you can even blink. So leap into health. Leap into confidence. Leap into sexy. Your body is ready for your journey, as winding and surprising as it may end up being. Your body is ready to heal, ready to grow, and ready to be sexy. And with love and support from me and the rest of the community of women behind you, you have even more power helping you stride joyfully forward.

Join us. Be your natural, sexy self. Live into a journey as full of uncertainty and surprises as it is of promises. Strut like you've got nothing to lose. You are an empowered, natural, sexy woman, and I welcome you to the roar.

Resources for Further Reading

Acne. Puusa, Seppo. *Clear for Life: Science-Based Natural Acne Treatment.* CreateSpace, 2013.

Autoimmune Healing. Ballantyne, Sarah. *The Paleo Approach: Reverse Autoimmune Disease, Heal Your Body.* Las Vegas: Victory Belt, 2014.

Baby and Child Care. Fallon Morell, Sally, and Thomas S. Cowan. *The Nourishing Traditions Book of Baby & Child Care.* Washington, D.C.: NewTrends, 2013.

Evolutionary Health. Jaminet, Paul, and Shou-Ching Jaminet. *Perfect Health Diet: Regain Health and Lose Weight by Eating the Way You Were Meant to Eat.* New York: Scribner, 2012.

Evolutionary Health. Trevathan, Wenda. *Ancient Bodies, Modern Lives: How Evolution Has Shaped Women's Health.* Oxford: Oxford University Press, 2001.

Evolutionary Health. Wolf, Robb. *The Paleo Solution: The Original Human Diet.* Las Vegas: Victory Belt, 2011.

Fertility Awareness Method. Weschler, Toni. *Taking Charge of Your Fertility: The Definitive Guide to Natural Birth Control, Pregnancy Achievement, and Reproductive Health.* New York: Collins, 2006.

Fitness. Shuler, Lou, Cassandra Forsythe, and Alwyn Cosgrove. *The New Rules of Lifting for Women: Lift Like a Man, Look Like a Goddess.* New York: Avery Trade, 2008.

Healthy Motherhood. Emch, Peggy. *Primal Moms Look Good Naked: A Mother's Guide to Achieving Beauty through Excellent Health.* Las Vegas: Victory Belt, 2013.

History. Diamond, Jared. *Guns, Germs, and Steel: The Fates of Human Societies.* New York: W. W. Norton, 2009.

Mental Health. Ross, Julia. *The Mood Cure: The 4-Step Program to Take Charge of Your Emotions—Today.* New York: Penguin, 2003.

Myth-Busting. Minger, Denise. *Death by Food Pyramid: How Shoddy Science, Sketchy Politics and Shady Special Interests Have Ruined Our Health.* Malibu, Calif.: Primal Nutrition, 2013.

Myth-Busting. Wolfe, Liz. *Eat the Yolks: Discover Paleo, Fight Food Lies, and Reclaim Your Health.* Las Vegas: Victory Belt, 2014.

Natural Childbirth. England, Pam, and Rob Horowitz. *Birthing from Within: An Extra-Ordinary Guide to Childbirth Preparation.* Albuquerque: Partera Press, 1998.

Natural Childbirth. Gaskin, Ina May. *Ina May's Guide to Childbirth.* New York: Bantam, 2003.

Vitamin D. Holick, Michael F. *The Vitamin D Solution: A 3-Step Strategy to Cure Our Most Common Health Problems.* New York: Plume, 2010.

Women and Fat. Lassek, William D., and Steven J. C. Gaulin. *Why Women Need Fat: How "Healthy" Food Makes Us Gain Excess Weight and the Surprising Solution to Losing It Forever.* New York: Hudson Street Press, 2011.

Resources for Natural Health and Lifestyle Implementation

Hartwig, Melissa, and Dallas Hartwig. *It Starts with Food: Discover the Whole30 and Change Your Life in Unexpected Ways.* Las Vegas: Victory Belt, 2012.

Sanfilippo, Diane. *Practical Paleo: A Customized Approach to Health and a Whole-Foods Lifestyle.* Las Vegas: Victory Belt, 2012.

Virgin, J. J. *The Virgin Diet: Drop 7 Foods, Lose 7 Pounds, Just 7 Days.* New York: Harlequin, 2012.

Resources for Cooking

Bauer, Juli, and George Bryant. *The Paleo Kitchen: Finding Primal Joy in Modern Cooking.* Las Vegas: Victory Belt, 2014.

Ciciarelli, Jill. *Fermented: A Four-Season Approach to Paleo Probiotic Foods.* Las Vegas: Victory Belt, 2013.

Joulwan, Melissa, and David Humphreys. *Well Fed: Paleo Recipes for People Who Love to Eat.* Austin, Tex.: Smudge, 2012.

McCarry, Matthew, and Stacy Toth. *Beyond Bacon: Paleo Recipes That Respect the Whole Hog.* Las Vegas: Victory Belt, 2013.

Staley, Bill, and Hayley Mason Staley. *Make It Paleo: Over 200 Grain-Free Recipes for Any Occasion.* Las Vegas: Victory Belt, 2011.

Tam, Michelle, and Henry Fong. *Nom Nom Paleo: Food for Humans.* Kansas City: Andrews McMeel, 2013.

Walker, Danielle. *Against All Grain: Delectable Paleo Recipes to Eat Well & Fell Great.* Las Vegas: Victory Belt, 2013.

Notes

[1] "The Facts about Diabetes: A Leading Cause of Death in the U.S.," *National Diabetes Education Program, Centers for Disease Control and Prevention,* accessed November 10, 2013, ndep.nih.gov/diabetes-facts.

[2] "Nutrition and Weight Management," *Boston Medical Center,* accessed Dec. 13, 2013, www.bmc.org/nutritionweight/services/weightmanagement.htm.

[3] "Vegetarianism in America," *Vegetarian Times,* accessed December 11, 2013. www.vegetariantimes.com/article/vegetarianism-in-america/.

[4] The China Study "conclusions" can be found in T. Colin Campbell's book *The China Study: The Most Comprehensive Study of Nutrition Ever Conducted* (New York: Bella Books, 2005). For a thorough analysis of the bias in Campbell's data analysis, see the work of Denise Minger at her website RawFoodSOS.com or in her book *Death by Food Pyramid: How Shoddy Science, Sketchy Politics and Shady Special Interests Have Ruined Our Health* (Malibu, Calif.: Primal Blueprint, 2013).

[5] These statistics are discussed at great length in David Kessler's book *The End of Overeating: Taking Control of the Insatiable American Appetite* (New York: Rodale, 2009).

[6] "Defining PCOS," *The University of Chicago: Medicine,* accessed December 10, 2013, www.uchospitals.edu/specialities/pcos/pcos.html.

[7] Sanjay Gupta, "If we are what we eat, Americans are corn and soy," *CNN,* accessed June 10, 2013, www.cnn.com/2007/HEALTH/diet.fitness/09/22/kd.gupta.column/.

[8] S. Lindeberg et al., "Palaeolithic diet improves glucose tolerance more than a Mediterranean-like diet in individuals with ischaemic heart disease," *Diabetologia* 50, no. 9 (2007), accessed December 10, 2013, www.springerlink.com/content/h7628r66r0552222.

[9] Joel Mason et al., "A Temporal Association between Folic Acid Fortification and an Increase in Colorectal Cancer Rates May Be Illuminating Important Biological Principles: A Hypothesis," *Cancer Epidemiology, Biomarkers & Prevention* 16 (July 2007): 1325–9, accessed December 1, 2013, cebp.aacrjournals.org/content/16/7/1325.

[10] Sarah Kobylewski and Michael F. Jacobson, "Food Dyes: A Rainbow of Risks," *Center for Science in the Public Interest,* June 2010, accessed December 10, 2013, cspinet.org/new/pdf/food-dyes-rainbow-of-risks.pdf.

[11] Jared Diamond, "The Worst Mistake in the History of the Human Race," *Discover Magazine,* May 1, 1987, 64–66, accessed June 10, 2013, www.zo.utexas.edu/courses/Thoc/Readings/Diamond_WorstMistake.pdf.

[12] Paul Jaminet and Shou-Ching Jaminet, *The Perfect Health Diet: Regain Health and Lose Weight by Eating the Way You Were Meant to Eat* (New York: Scribner, 2012), 115. Data from Stephan Guyenet, "Seed oils and body fatness—a problematic revisit," blog post, August 21, 2011, wholehealthsource.blogspot.com/2011/08/seed-oils-and-body-fatness-problematic.html.

[13] Jaminet and Jaminet discuss these statistics at length in the section on seed oils in their book *The Perfect Health Diet*.

[14] A. P. Simopoulous, "The Importance of the Ratio of Omega 6/Omega 3 Essential Fatty Acids," *Biomedical Pharmaceuticals* 56, no. 8 (October 2002): 365–79.

[15] Chris Kresser, "Liver: Nature's Most Potent Superfood," April 2008, accessed December 10, 2013, chriskresser.com/natures-most-potent-superfood.

[16] H. Petursson et al., "Is the Use of Cholesterol in Mortality Risk Algorithms in Clinical Guidelines Valid? Ten Years Prospective Data from the Norwegian HUNT 2 Study," *Journal of Evaluation of Clinical Practice* 1 (February 2012): 159–68.

[17] Carolyn Coker Ross, "Why Do Women Hate Their Bodies?," *PsychCentral*, 2012, accessed December 12, 2013, psychcentral.com/blog/archives/2012/06/02/why-do-women-hate-their-bodies.

[18] "Sedentary Lives Can Be Deadly: Physical Inactivity Poses Greatest Health Risk to Americans, Experts Say," *Science Daily*, August 10, 2009, accessed June 24, 2013, www.sciencedaily.com/releases/2009/08/090810024825.htm.

[19] Terry Boyle, Lin Fritschi, Jane Heyworth, and Fiona Bull, "Long-Term Sedentary Work and the Risk of Subsite-specific Colorectal Cancer," *American Journal of Epidemiology* (2011), accessed December 12, 2013, aje.oxfordjournals.org/content/early/2011/03/18/aje.kwq513.abstract. See also Brigid M. Lynch, "Sedentary Behavior and Cancer: A Systematic Review of the Literature and Proposed Biological Mechanisms," *Cancer, Epidemiology, Biomarkers, & Prevention* 19 (November 2010): 2692 and William Hudson, "Sitting for hours can shave years off life," *CNN*, June 24, 2011, accessed December 12, 2013, www.cnn.com/2011/HEALTH/06/24/sitting.shorten.life/index.html.

[20] Andrew Hough, "30 minutes exercise 'better than an hour of training' for weight loss," *The Telegraph*, August 2012, accessed August 20, 2013, www.telegraph.co.uk/health/healthnews/9493863/30-minutes-exercise-better-than-an-hour-of-training-for-weight-loss.html.

[21] Valerie Gaudreault et al., "Transient Myocardial Tissue and Function Changes During a Marathon in Less Fit Marathon Runners," *Canadian Journal of Cardiology* 29, no. 10 (October 2013): 1269–76.

[22] T. Shiraev, "Evidence based exercise—clinical benefits of high intensity interval training," *Australian Family Physicians* 12 (2012): 960–2.

[23] Gary Small, "Can Exercise Cure Depression?," *Psychology Today* (September 2010), accessed Dec. 10, 2013, www.psychologytoday.com/blog/brain-bootcamp/201009/can-exercise-cure-depression.

[24] Wesley J. Wildman, *Science and Religious Anthropology: A Spiritually Evocative Naturalist Interpretation of Human Life* (Farnham: Ashgate, 2009).

[25] Anjani Chandra, Casey Copehn, and Elizabeth Hervey Stephen, "Infertility and Impaired Fecundity in the United States, 1982–2010: Data from the National Survey of Family Growth," *National Health Statistics Reports* 67 (August 14, 2013).

[26] "Defining PCOS," *The University of Chicago: Medicine,* accessed December 10, 2013, www.uchospitals.edu/specialitites/pcos/pcos.html.

[27] C. A. Shivley, "Social stress, visceral obesity, and coronary artery atherosclerosis: product of a primate adaptation," *American Journal of Primatology* 71, no. 9 (2009): 742–51.

[28] For a more in-depth discussion of body fatness, leptin, development, and fertility, see Wenda Trevathan, *Ancient Bodies, Modern Lives: How Evolution Has Shaped Women's Health* (Oxford: Oxford University Press, 2001), 28–30.

[29] "The Birth Control Pill—A History," *Katharine Dexter McCormick Library* and *Planned Parenthood Federation of America* (April 2010), accessed December 10, 2013, www.plannedparenthood.org/files/PPFA/PPFA_ib_Pill_Ann_051010.pdf.

[30] Mohamed M. Ali et al., "Long-term Contraceptive Protection, Discontinuation and Switching Behavior: Intrauterine Device Use Dynamics in 14 Developing Countries," *World Health Organization and Marie Stopes International,* 2011, accessed December 10, 2013, www.who.int/reproductivehealth/publications/family_planning/Long_term_contraceptive_protection_behaviour.pdf.

[31] Edward Laumann, Anthony Paik, and Raymond Rosen, "Sexual Dysfunction in the United States: Prevalence and Predictors," *Journal of the American Medical Association* 281, no. 6 (February 1999): 537–44.

[32] "How Many People Are Affected by or at Risk for Endometriosis?," *Eunice Kennedy Shriver National Institute of Child Health and Human Development,* 2011, accessed December 10, 2013, www.nichd.nih.gov/health/topics/endometri/conditioninfo/pages/at-risk.aspx.

[33] Jennifer Daw, "Is PMDD Real? Researchers, Physicians, and Psychologists Fall on Various Sides of the Debate over Premenstrual Dysphoric Disorder," *American Psychological Association* 33, no. 9 (2002): 58.

[34] J. A. Blumenthal et al., "Effects of Exercise Training on Older Patients with Major Depression," *Archives of Internal Medicine* 159, no. 19 (1999): 2349–56.

Index

5-HTP, food cravings and, 149

A
abdominal fat, 223
acceptance, 40, 195
acne, 230
  bacteria and, 234
  birth control pills and, 233
  blood sugar and, 231
  gut health and, 233–234
  inflammation and, 233–234
  insulin resistance and, 231
  menstrual cycle and, 232–233
  starvation and, 232
  touching skin and, 236
addictive quality of foods, food industry
  and, 56
adrenal glands, 210
  caffeine and, 159
  infertility and, 256
  sleep and, 207
advertising, 56–58
affirmation, need for, 312–313
aging, 239–240. *See also* menopause
  attitude and, 241
  fasting and, 240–241
  grandmothers, 242
  low-carbohydrate diet, 241
  nourishment and, 240
  sleep and, 168
agriculture, human health and, 102
alcohol
  inflammation and, 85
  sugar and, 97
allergies
  dairy and, 130–131
  gut bacteria and, 80
alone time, 305
Alzheimer's disease, inflammation
  and, 84
amino acids, 90
  grains, 100–101
animal fats, industrialization and, 122
animal protein, 90, 114
  animals' diets, 122
    dairy and, 131
  beef, 120
  necessity of, 34–35
  organ meat, 121, 123

sources, 35
vitamins, 34–35
antibodies, sleep and, 168
antioxidants, skin and, 237
anxiety, 278–280
  inflammation and, 84
appetite, leptin and, 88–89
arthritis, inflammation and, 84
asceticism, 29
  blame on hearty foods, 33
  fasting, 30
  low-calorie dieting, 31–32
  low-fat dieting, 32–33
  women and, 30–31
asthma
  gut bacteria and, 80
  inflammation and, 84
autoimmune disease, 83
  gut bacteria and, 80
avocado oil, 126–127

B
bacteria, acne and, 234
basal metabolic rate, strength/weight
  training and, 179
beans, 104–105. *See also* legumes
beauty conformity, 25–26
beauty products, 28
beef, benefits, 119–120
beets, 117
beta-carotene, 80
beverages, 96
birth control. *See also* hormonal birth
  control; non-hormonal birth control
  acne and, 233
  hormone imbalance and, 233
  infertility and, 254–255
  weight and, 223–224
blood pressure
  cortisol and, 156
  sex and, 185
blood sugar
  acne, 231
  alcohol, 97
  breakfast, 142
  carbohydrates and, 137–138
  cortisol and, 156
  energy and, 214–215
  fruit and, 118